Navigating Cardiology's Future

Amir Ghaffari Jolfayi
Editor

Sanaz Asadian • Golnaz Houshmand
Associate Editors

Navigating Cardiology's Future

AI in MRI Imaging and Outcome Projections

Springer

Editor
Amir Ghaffari Jolfayi
Cardiovascular Imaging Research Center
Rajaie Cardiovascular Institute
Tehran, Iran

Associate Editors
Sanaz Asadian
Department of Radiology
Cardiothoracic Imaging Section
University of Washington
Seattle, USA

Golnaz Houshmand
Cardiovascular Imaging Research Center
Rajaie Cardiovasular Institute
Tehran, Iran

ISBN 978-981-95-0312-4 ISBN 978-981-95-0313-1 (eBook)
https://doi.org/10.1007/978-981-95-0313-1

This Springer imprint is published by the registered company Springer Nature Singapore Pte Ltd.
The registered company address is: 152 Beach Road, #21-01/04 Gateway East, Singapore 189721, Singapore

Preface

The field of cardiology is undergoing a seismic shift, propelled by artificial intelligence and advanced imaging technologies. *Navigating Cardiology's Future* was born from a pressing need to consolidate the latest advancements in AI-powered cardiac MRI and outcome prediction into a single, accessible resource. This book bridges the gap between theoretical AI algorithms and their real-world clinical applications, offering insights that are both scientifically rigorous and practically relevant.

Why is this book important? Because AI is no longer a futuristic concept—it is here, transforming how we diagnose, monitor, and predict cardiovascular diseases. Whether you are a cardiologist seeking to integrate AI into your practice, a researcher exploring machine learning in medical imaging, or a technologist developing the next generation of diagnostic tools, this book provides the knowledge you need to navigate this evolving landscape.

The chapters span the historical evolution of cardiac imaging, the fundamentals of AI and deep learning, and their applications across various cardiac conditions—cardiomyopathy, coronary artery disease, arrhythmias, and inflammatory heart disease. A dedicated SWOT analysis evaluates the strengths, weaknesses, opportunities, and threats of AI in cardiology, while the final chapter explores AI-driven risk stratification for cardiovascular outcomes.

This project would not have been possible without the support of numerous colleagues, mentors, and institutions. We extend our deepest gratitude to the Professors of radiology, cardiology, computer science, and medical doctors, residents, and cardiac imaging fellows, whose expertise, collaboration, and dedication were instrumental in the conception and preparation of this book.

We hope this book serves as both a guide and an inspiration, empowering readers to harness the full potential of AI in advancing cardiovascular care.

Tehran, Iran — Amir Ghaffari Jolfayi
Seattle, USA — Sanaz Asadian
Tehran, Iran — Golnaz Houshmand

Acknowledgments

This book is the culmination of years of research, collaboration, and shared expertise, and we owe immense gratitude to the many individuals and institutions who made it possible.

First and foremost, we extend our deepest appreciation to the Department of Radiology at Rajaie Cardiovascular Medical and Research Center for their unwavering support, resources, and encouragement throughout this project. Our colleagues and fellow researchers in Cardiovascular Imaging at Rajaie Institute have been instrumental in shaping the clinical and technical perspectives presented in this work.

We are also profoundly grateful to the Department of Radiology at UW Medicine, Seattle, United States, particularly post-doctoral researchers whose groundbreaking research in AI and cardiac imaging inspired the discussions in this book. Their mentorship and collaboration have been invaluable.

Special thanks go to the faculty members, professors and radiology residents, fellows, medical imaging PhD students, and scholars who contributed through insightful discussions, case studies, and technical feedback. Their dedication to advancing cardiovascular imaging fuels the future of this field.

Finally, we acknowledge the countless researchers, clinicians, and engineers worldwide whose pioneering work in AI and MRI continues to push the boundaries of cardiology. This book stands on the shoulders of their innovations.

To all who supported this endeavor, thank you.

Tehran, Iran — Amir Ghaffari Jolfayi
Seattle, USA — Sanaz Asadian
Tehran, Iran — Golnaz Houshmand

About the Book

Cardiology stands at the precipice of a revolution, one driven by the rapid advancements in artificial intelligence and magnetic resonance imaging. *Navigating Cardiology's Future: AI in MRI Imaging and Outcome Projections* is a timely and essential exploration of how these technologies are reshaping diagnostic precision, prognostic accuracy, and therapeutic decision-making in cardiovascular medicine.

The integration of AI into cardiac MRI has unlocked unprecedented capabilities—enhancing image analysis, automating complex measurements, and uncovering patterns invisible to the human eye. This book meticulously examines these innovations, offering clinicians, researchers, and technologists a comprehensive guide to the present and future of AI-driven cardiology.

As someone who has witnessed the evolution of cardiac imaging firsthand, I am deeply impressed by the depth and clarity with which this book addresses both foundational concepts and cutting-edge applications. From cardiomyopathy to coronary artery disease, arrhythmias to inflammatory heart conditions, the authors provide a roadmap for leveraging AI to improve patient outcomes.

This is not just a book—it is an invitation to embrace the transformative potential of AI in cardiology. I wholeheartedly recommend it to anyone invested in the future of cardiovascular care.

Amir Ghaffari Jolfayi
Spring 2025

Contents

The Evolution of Cardiac Imaging: From Radiography to Feature Tracking and T1/T2 Mapping Analysis in Cardiac Magnetic Resonance Imaging

1

Amir Azimi, Hadis Ehsandoust,
Mohammadhossein Mozafarybazargany,
Sanaz Asadian, Hamidreza Ghasemirad,
Msoumeh Ahmadi, and Amir Ghaffari Jolfayi

Abstract

Cardiac imaging has undergone a remarkable transformation, evolving from early X-ray techniques to sophisticated cardiovascular magnetic resonance (CMR) imaging, which now plays a critical role in diagnosing and managing heart diseases. This review highlights the historical development, technological breakthroughs, and clinical applications of cardiac imaging, with a focus on the impact of CMR.

Initial efforts in cardiac imaging relied on basic X-rays and fluoroscopy, offering limited diagnostic capabilities. Innovations such as orthodiagraphy and roentgen cinematography advanced the ability to measure cardiac dimensions and motion. The mid-twentieth century saw significant progress with cardiac angiography and coronary arteriography, enabling detailed visualization of heart anatomy and pathology. The introduction of iodinated and non-iodinated contrast media further refined these methods, paving the way for modern imaging techniques. The emergence of echocardiography and nuclear imaging expanded the assessment of cardiac function and perfusion.

CMR has become a cornerstone of advanced cardiac imaging, offering exceptional capabilities in tissue characterization, functional assessment, and diagnosis without ionizing radiation. Techniques like T1 and T2 mapping quantify myocardial tissue properties such as fibrosis, edema, and infiltration, providing early insights into disease processes. T2* mapping has emerged as a valuable tool for assessing myocardial iron overload and detecting hemorrhage. Late gadolinium enhancement (LGE), a hallmark of CMR, identifies and quantifies myocardial fibrosis with unparalleled spatial resolution, enabling precise differentiation between ischemic and non-ischemic patterns of scarring. Strain analysis using feature tracking quantifies myocardial deforma-

Authors Amir Azimi and Hadis Ehsandoust have contributed equality and shared the first co-authorship.

A. Azimi · H. Ehsandoust · M. Mozafarybazargany
M. Ahmadi · A. Ghaffari Jolfayi (✉)
Cardiovascular Imaging Research Center, Rajaie Cardiovascular Institute, Iran University of Medical Sciences, Tehran, Iran

S. Asadian
Department of Radiology, Cardiothoracic Imaging, University of Washington, Seattle, USA

H. Ghasemirad
Student Research Committee, Shahid Sadoughi University of Medical Sciences, Yazd, Iran

A. Ghaffari Jolfayi (ed.), *Navigating Cardiology's Future*,
https://doi.org/10.1007/978-981-95-0313-1_1

tion, enhancing early detection of subclinical dysfunction and risk stratification.

Recent advancements in CMR include 4D imaging, diffusion-weighted imaging for detailed tissue characterization, and advanced respiratory and cardiac gating for superior image quality. Artificial Intelligence integration is further transforming CMR through faster acquisition, enhanced interpretation, and improved predictive modeling. These innovations solidify CMR's role in personalized cardiac care, offering unprecedented diagnostic and prognostic capabilities. Future developments, such as feature tracking for strain analysis and Artificial Intelligence integration, promise to enhance the precision and utility of CMR further. This review provides a comprehensive overview of the evolution of cardiac imaging, emphasizing its pivotal role in advancing cardiovascular care and shaping future clinical practices.

Keywords

Cardiac magnetic resonance imaging · Radiography · Computed tomography imaging · Coronary computed tomography angiography · T1/T2 mapping analysis · Feature tracking · Deep learning · Machine learning · Artificial Intelligence

1.1 From Early X-Ray to Advanced MRI

1.1.1 Overview of Cardiac Imaging

The term "cardiac imaging" describes several methods developed over time to study the structure and function of the heart [1]. Using these techniques, medical professionals can identify and track cardiac conditions such as congenital heart abnormalities, cardiomyopathies, and coronary artery disease [2].

1.1.2 Imaging's Significance in Heart Care

This passage from one of the most important books of the twentieth century describes the amazement and fascination people felt when they used fluoroscopy to see how the heart moved. Throughout the first half of the twentieth century, imaging played a minimal role in diagnosing and managing heart diseases. The most well-known early twentieth-century cardiology textbooks in this era devoted only a brief chapter to cardiac imaging, often shorter than the one on electrocardiography, or did not address cardiac imaging [3, 4]. At the time, three roentgenology techniques were available: teleroentgenography, fluoroscopy, and orthodiagraphy; this method required tracing cardiac images onto transparent sheets positioned on a fluoroscopy screen. Four heart views were available with teleroentgenography, often known as radiography: frontal, lateral, right anterior oblique, and left anterior oblique.

In some ways, White minimizes the importance of roentgenology at this point, saying, "It must be acknowledged that serious heart disease may exist or be found in other ways when roentgenology does not reveal its presence." Therefore, roentgenology typically only shows signs of a well-established illness that is hard or impossible to treat [5, 6]. Thus, at the beginning of the twentieth century, most well-known cardiologists acknowledged that cardiac imaging had minimal application. However, in the 1930s, two full textbooks were available that explained how radiography could be used to show the normal and pathological appearance of the heart [7, 8]. Before 1950, a few radiology publications showed some cardiac imaging innovations. Still, they did not hint at the significant role cardiac imaging would play in the proceeding decades of the twentieth century [8].

1.1.3 Early Heart Imaging Years

In a 1925 lecture to the Radiological Society of North America, Hodges emphasized the diagnostic value of heart measurements obtained through radiographic and fluoroscopic methods. He highlighted the need to account for factors like age, body size, and other variables when assessing cardiac dimensions and stressed the importance of indexing these measurements. Tables outlining standard cardiac sizes for fluoroscopy and frontal radiography were also noted as reference tools [9, 10]. Eisen's paper emphasized the importance of using a frontal chest radiograph taken during full inspiration for accurately assessing heart size and shape. At a time when chest radiographs were the primary imaging option, roentgen cinematography was employed to capture heart motion, producing 15 frontal radiographs per second [11]. A method known as roentgen cinematography was used to record cardiac motion from the frontal perspective. Using this method, 15 frontal radiographs could be taken per second, and each radiograph's location in the cardiac cycle could be referenced simultaneously. This was a primitive technique for observing and documenting cardiac rhythms [5].

The method of recording myocardial contraction on a frontal radiograph provided limited information due to its focus on the ventricle contour. Orthodiagraphy was developed to enhance the accuracy and consistency of heart size measurements by reducing magnification artifacts resulting from divergent X-rays in the frontal projection. This method outlines opaque shadows in their actual size by utilizing a narrow, collimated portion of the fluoroscopic X-ray beam [12, 13]. The resulting orthodiagraphic tracings were significantly smaller than the heart's shadow as seen on a standard fluoroscopic screen. Hodges and Eyster determined that if the measured cardiac silhouette area exceeded the predicted area—adjusted for age, body size, and heart rate—by 7% or more, there was a threefold likelihood of cardiac disease [12–14]. Rigler's article highlighted the importance of left atrial enlargement on lateral radiographs to differentiate between heart lesions and mitral valve disease [14]. He proposed that congenital cardiac defects and pulmonary abnormalities lead to heart enlargement but not esophagus compression or displacement. This was the first article to propose evaluating the left atrium in the differential diagnosis of cardiomegaly. Later, Roentgen kymography was used to characterize pulmonary arterial pulsations.

Cross-sectional cardiac radiography was investigated in 1939, laying the groundwork for the development of advanced cross-sectional cardiac imaging technologies in subsequent decades. Two methods were used: the first involved capturing a single radiograph with the central ray entering the upper dorsal spine of a forward-tilting body and exiting at the sternodiaphragmatic angle. The second method involved rotating the patient 360° around the vertical axis while recording the cardiac borders across various diameters, allowing for reconstructing a cross-sectional image of the heart [5].

1.2 X-Ray (Radiography) and Fluoroscopy

1.2.1 The Emergence of X-Rays for Cardiac Imaging

The invention of kymography allowed for recording ventricular border movements throughout the cardiac cycle [15]. The process entailed projecting the edge of the heart onto a film that had a horizontal slit to project X-rays onto it. Later, the method was applied to determine the approximate boundaries of the end diastole and systole [16]. It was used to assess regional impairments in myocardial function occurring in acute and chronic infarctions of the myocardium, as well as cardiac output and aortic flexibility [17].

1.2.2 Cardiac Angiography

Robb and Steinberg in the United States and Castellanos et al. in Cuba were the pioneers in the introduction and promotion of intravenous cardio angiography. To get single or serial radiographs, the approach entailed that iodinated contrast media be manually injected vigorously into one or more antecubital veins [18, 19]. The sequential opacification from the superior vena cava to the pulmonary circulation was displayed. These studies provided the first in vivo visualization of the anatomy of specific congenital heart abnormalities [18, 19], one of the abnormalities was tetralogy of Fallot [20]. Serial radiography was also utilized to explore the pathoanatomy of the left side of the heart in various acquired cardiac diseases [20–22]. However, this technique produced suboptimal opacification of the left-sided chambers. For accurate diagnosis of congenital and acquired cardiovascular lesions on the left side, selective catheterization of both the right and left sides of the heart would be necessary [22]. Significant advancements in cardiac angiography were made with the introduction of selective conventional angiography and biplane cine angiocardiography, enabling detailed diagnosis of acquired and congenital cardiac lesions [22–24].

1.2.3 Coronary Arteriography

Direct coronary artery visualization was developed over three decades using various experimental techniques [23–25]. In the early 1960s, cardiac diagnosticians achieved direct coronary catheterization using occlusion aortography in dogs. The selective catheterization of coronary arteries, facilitating the advent of coronary angiography in humans, was accomplished in the mid-1960s. Judkins' technique revolutionized the diagnosis and treatment of coronary artery disease by using preshaped catheters for the right and left coronary arteries. Other methods used catheters designed to conform to the sinuses of Valsalva [23].

1.2.4 Cardiac Angiography Application

From 1950 to 1980, Radiology described radiographic and angiographic diagnostic features for various cardiovascular lesions, including Takayasu arteritis, constrictive pericardial disease, thoracic aortic dissection, and radiation-induced heart disease. Angiographic findings during this period aided in diagnosis, influenced prognosis, and provided critical insights into coronary arterial anomalies [26].

Iodinated and Non-iodinated Contrast Media Before introducing non-iodinated contrast media, iodinated contrast media were used extensively. After extensive investigations, cardiotoxic effects of ionic iodinated contrast media, causing temporary cardiac dysfunction, ventricular arrhythmias, and reduction of heart rate, were revealed. Consequently, the development of modern nonionic iodinated contrast media focused on achieving an ideal balance of composition and osmolality [27–29].

1.2.5 Cardiac Ultrasound

Advancements in cardiac ultrasonography introduced the use of indocyanine green solution to improve the visualization of cardiac anatomy and function, building on its existing applications in detecting structural heart abnormalities, mitral valve disease, and pericardial effusion, thereby broadening its diagnostic capabilities [30, 31]. Echocardiography has emerged as the preferred noninvasive imaging modality in cardiology given its diverse advanced modes, including 3D imaging, strain tracking, speckle tracking analysis, Doppler imaging, and novel applications and methods like intracardiac and portable US. The standards of the effective utilization of echocardiography, professional requirements, and essential training have all been established [32, 33].

1.2.6 Nuclear Medicine Imaging

The Radiology published a study in 1974 on nuclear medicine techniques to illustrate a myocardial infarction [34, 35]. Technetium 99 m stannous pyrophosphate was first utilized to demonstrate myocardial infarction because of the initial discovery that mitochondria of cardiac cells experiencing permanent cell damage following ischemia accumulate calcium ions. In irreversibly damaged cardiac cells, the radionuclide tracer binds to the crystalline structure of hydroxyapatite, where calcium ions are concentrated within the mitochondria, a process commonly referred to as "hot spot" imaging. Subsequent studies highlighted the potential of magnetic resonance imaging (MRI) and computed tomography (CT) in detecting acute myocardial infarction, building on the foundation laid by these early investigations. In addition, it was demonstrated that rubidium 81 has advantageous properties for human cardiac perfusion scanning [35]. This radioisotope has been effectively used for both resting and stress myocardial perfusion imaging, also known as "dark spot" imaging. By integrating markers of blood flow and glucose uptake, positron emission tomography (PET) was first described in the journal in the 1970s to assess cardiac tissue viability [36]. While viability was determined by maintaining glucose utilization (or "mismatch") in hypoperfused myocardial segments at rest, concordant declines in segmental glucose utilization and perfusion were defined as myocardial infarction (MI) ("matched defect"). These days, patients suspected of having coronary artery disease (CAD) can be evaluated using nuclear medicine techniques such as single photon emission computed tomography (SPECT) and PET, which use myocardial perfusion imaging. Compared to SPECT myocardial perfusion, PET myocardial perfusion has a higher sensitivity and spatial resolution [37]. Moreover, myocardial vitality and neoangiogenesis, matrix metalloproteinase activity, and sympathetic cardiac innervation are all revealed by SPECT and PET imaging [37]. Integration of imaging systems is a recent trend in cardiac imaging. For instance, hybrid cardiac imaging with fluorine-18 fluorodeoxyglucose PET on an integrated PET/MR system allows for assessing myocardial viability in patients with infarcts by combining glucose imaging with late gadolinium-enhanced (LGE) imaging [38].

1.2.7 Cardiac CT

In 1980, cardiac CT became a clinical tool. From the start, the use of electrocardiographically gated cardiac CT proved useful in showcasing a variety of diseases, including thrombus, enhanced scars, and left ventricular aneurysms [39]. It was quickly acknowledged and documented that CT could diagnose aortic dissection [39]. Recent studies focused on coronary artery disease emphasize the use of CT and MR imaging in diagnosis and management [40].

Coronary Calcifications It has long been acknowledged that showcasing coronary calcifications is a significant CT application. A substantial negative predictive value for clinically severe CAD was found when coronary calcifications were absent on CT [41]. Technical considerations were found to be crucial in ensuring the consistent and reliable imaging of coronary calcifications [42]. High correlations were seen when estimations of coronary calcifications were validated using electron-beam CT versus histomorphometry. Moreover, a strong correlation was observed between the quantity of calcific deposits and the degree of coronary stenosis. Comparing the volumetric score to the conventional Agatston score has improved repeatability [43]. In addition, the effect of calcium measurement and scanner type has been assessed to estimate the reproducibility of calcium scores. The results of multi-detector row and electron-beam CT scans showed similar repeatability when assessing coronary calcium. The reproducibility of calcium volume estimates was marginally higher than that of Agatston scores [43]. A large cohort of asymptomatic individuals underwent electron-beam CT analysis to assess the prognostic value of coronary calcium scores. This study demonstrated that the coronary calcium score provides independent and incremental predictive value for all-cause mortality beyond traditional risk factors [44]. Furthermore, large population-based cohort studies have effectively implemented and produced consistent results at numerous sites when measuring coronary calcifications using cardiac-gated CT [45].

1.2.8 Coronary CT Angiography

After coronary CT angiography was developed, clinical indications quickly advanced, with multi-detector row CT angiography emerging as a reliable method for identifying vessel origin and course in patients suspected of coronary anomalies. Improvements in multi-detector row CT technology, which offered shorter acquisition times, necessitated refining contrast material injection protocols to ensure precise synchronization between contrast passage and cardiac image acquisition [46–48].

Despite challenges related to calcifications and motion artifacts, CT technology has advanced rapidly, significantly improving its diagnostic capabilities for detecting CAD. Meta-analyses revealed that 64-section spiral CT offered substantially higher specificity and positive predictive value per patient compared to earlier generations of multidetector CT for identifying coronary artery stenosis exceeding 50%. However, the widespread adoption of coronary CT angiography also brought increased attention to the radiation doses associated with the procedure [49].

Several CT techniques have been developed to evaluate the functional significance of CAD, including CT angiography combined with fractional flow reserve analysis, myocardial perfusion imaging, and assessment of diffuse coronary artery disease using scaling power laws. Multicenter trials have demonstrated that incorporating coronary CT angiography into the diagnostic approach for patients with acute chest pain and suspected acute coronary syndromes is both safe and effective. This approach enhances clinical decision-making and facilitates faster discharge from the emergency department [50].

1.2.9 Myocardial Perfusion Imaging

Following gadopentetate dimeglumine injection, first-pass myocardial perfusion imaging is now possible thanks to ultrafast T1-weighted MR sequences [51]. This approach outperforms SPECT imaging regarding diagnostic accuracy for identifying severe coronary artery disease. When black-blood T2-weighted inversion-recovery MR imaging was first introduced, it was possible to see low-intensity areas within the infarcted region that may have been caused by postreperfusion hemorrhage in addition to areas of infarction with high signal intensity due to edema. The area at risk and hemorrhage can now be shown using T2-weighted MR techniques as indicators of the severity of cardiac injury [51, 52].

1.3 The Emergence of MRI: A Game-Changer in Cardiology

Various imaging techniques are used to assess cardiac and pericardial lesions, each with distinct benefits and limitations. Transthoracic echocardiography, widely accessible, is the preferred method for diagnosing intracardiac lesions, offering insights into the size, movement, shape, and position of cardiac masses. However, it lacks detailed information on tissue characteristics. For specific patient groups, such as those with chronic obstructive pulmonary disease or obesity, transesophageal echocardiography serves as an alternative diagnostic option [53, 54]. Cardiovascular CT is a noninvasive imaging technique that provides high spatial and adequate temporal resolution. It enables visualization of cardiac and intracardiac masses, facilitating the evaluation of their involvement in the heart and pericardium. However, the procedure requires exposure to radiation and the use of an iodinated contrast agent, which limits its application [55].

Cardiac magnetic resonance (CMR) offers numerous advantages in diagnosing cardiac lesions. CMR accurately characterizes tissue composition through intrinsic T1 and T2 relaxation analysis, unlike other imaging modalities. It also provides a wide field of view, superior temporal and spatial resolution, 3D multiplanar imaging, and the ability to assess lymph node inflammation, the mediastinum, and adjacent vascular structures [56, 57]. CMR is a crucial imaging tool for diagnosing cardiac malignancies, offering a comprehensive evaluation of anatomy, functionality, tissue composition, vascularity, and interactions with surrounding tissues. It is particularly valuable for detecting prior malignancies in cases of cardiac metastases and identifying metastatic lesions in the chest, liver, or abdomen [58].

Recent advancements in noninvasive imaging techniques have significantly improved the functional evaluation of coronary artery disease (CAD). Key approaches include stress perfusion imaging, dobutamine stress cardiac magnetic resonance imaging (MRI), and stress echocardiography. Among these, modalities such as MRI, CT, PET, and SPECT have become the most widely used methods for assessing coronary artery stenosis [59].

Newly developed PET-MRI hybrid scanners integrate the strengths of both PET and MRI, offering advanced clinical imaging capabilities. In this context, cardiac MR stress perfusion imaging stands out as the primary MRI technique for evaluating cardiac stress [58].

In recent years, CMR has been increasingly used as a diagnostic and risk classification tool for patients with heart disease. It is widely regarded as the most efficient and reliable method for noninvasively assessing the volume and function of the ventricles, evaluating the viability of the heart muscle, and determining the properties of biological tissues [59–62].

1.3.1 Morphologic MR Imaging

Since the 1970s, scientists have used radionuclides, iodinated contrast agents, and magnetic resonance contrast agents to visualize myocardial infarction following ischemia noninvasively [63, 64]. CT, in combination with iodinated contrast media in experimental work, is where the history of contrast media for cardiac imaging started [64]. Afterward, it was determined that some characteristics of myocardial contrast enhancement in infarcted regions held significant clinical relevance based on initial research. In an animal model, manganese was employed as an MR contrast agent to distinguish between normal and ischemic myocardium; however, its toxicity limited its practical utility [65]. The ability of other MR contrast agents, such as gadopentetate dimeglumine, to detect acute myocardial ischemia has been studied [66]. In addition to being useful in describing other cardiac disorders like myocarditis, LGE has emerged as one of the main benefits of MRI for diagnosing ischemia and nonischemic cardiomyopathies [67, 68]. Modified wideband LGE MRI has been presented recently, which allows diagnostic imaging of cardiac scars in patients with implanted cardiac devices by removing hyperintensity artifacts from implanted devices [68]. Cardiovascular molecular MR imaging techniques, serial myocardial R1 (1/T1) mapping, myocardial T1 mapping, and other new MR techniques are being extensively investigated for improved cardiac tissue characterization [69–71].

1.3.2 Functional MR Imaging

The left ventricular mass has been highly accurately and consistently estimated by MR imaging [72, 73]. Cine MR approaches have been developed for functional cardiac imaging, including regurgitant fraction estimation in patients with regurgitant mitral and aortic valve disease. Steady-state free precession MR imaging enhances blood-myocardium contrast, resulting in higher left ventricular volume estimates. Additionally, myocardial tagging using MR imaging has been presented, offering information on heart motion and permitting the assessment of myocardial deformation in three dimensions [74, 75].

1.3.3 Coronary MR Angiography

Currently, CT and MRI, with MRI playing a more limited role, are used for noninvasive coronary artery imaging. Initial reports on breath-hold MR angiography emerged, demonstrating its reliability in visualizing segments of the proximal coronary arteries in healthy individuals [76]. Parts of the coronary arteries could be seen after multiplanar reconstruction was applied to a volume of images. Even though the technology was still in its infancy, two-dimensional coronary MR angiography exhibited a relatively low sensitivity for identifying hemodynamically severe coronary artery stenosis. Real-time respiratory gating and triggering based on navigator echo were implemented to increase the dependability of coronary MR angiography. This strategy reduced breathing artifacts during coronary MR angiographic acquisitions realistically and efficiently. Navigation technology was modified to increase the speed and quality of coronary MR image acquisition. Using broader gating windows and prospective adaptive navigators to adjust image positioning during free-breathing coronary MR angiography effectively decreases the overall imaging duration while maintaining image quality comparable to breath-hold coronary MR angiography. For three-dimensional coronary magnetic resonance angiography, placing the navigator at the right hemidiaphragm was favored over positioning it at the left ventricle. Heart and breathing motion continued to be a persistent problem for coronary magnetic resonance imaging acquisition strategies that aim to account for this motion. According to a prospective multicenter investigation, three-dimensional coronary MR angiography is reliable in ruling out coronary artery stenosis in or out within the proximal and middle segments. A navigator-gated steady-state sequence in whole-heart coronary MR angiography was suggested to enhance imaging of all three major coronary arteries [77–79].

According to a multicenter investigation, patients with coronary artery disease can be accurately diagnosed with severe coronary artery stenosis using nonenhanced whole-heart coronary MR angiography. According to the study, whole-heart coronary MR angiography at 1.5 T had an 88% negative predictive value, high sensitivity, and moderate specificity [80]. The development of more accurate cardiovascular function measurements and the incorporation of imaging methods into interventional treatments have resulted from this breakthrough in imaging technologies and improved patient care [79, 80].

1.4 The Evolution of MRI Sequences and Novel Techniques in Cardiology

Over the past 50 years, cardiovascular magnetic resonance (CMR) has emerged as a powerful non-invasive imaging modality without ionizing radiation. Its development evolved through clinical use origins, CMR-specific techniques advancement, and integration into cardiovascular care pathways [81, 82]. During the second stage, spanning the 1980s to 2010, investigators harnessed CMR's capabilities to assess cardiovascular anatomy, cardiac motion and deformation, myocardial perfusion, blood flow, and metabolism. Crucially, they developed techniques such as T1, T2, and T2* mapping to characterize myocardial tissue at the voxel level, quantifying edema, fibrosis, infiltration (e.g., amyloid), and LGE for infarct/thrombus detection [81, 83].

With these innovations, the third stage from 2010 onward has seen widespread clinical adoption of comprehensive CMR protocols. By combining its multiparametric features, CMR provides unprecedented insights into cardiovascular disease processes, aiding diagnosis, monitoring, and management strategies for improved patient care [82, 84]. This section focuses on two essential techniques: LGE and tissue characterization techniques such as T1, T2, T2*, and extracellular volume (ECV) mapping, evaluating their roles as diagnostic and prognostic tools.

1.4.1 Late Gadolinium Enhancement (LGE)

LGE is a CMR technique used for tissue characterization [85]. The LGE technique involves acquiring images 10–20 min after injecting a gadolinium-based contrast agent (0.1–0.2 mmol/Kg). Gadolinium is an extracellular contrast agent that exits blood vessels and spreads into the interstitial space after intravenous injection. It is routinely used in MRI due to its T1-shortening solid effect and tissue-dependent distribution within the body. In normal myocardium, gadolinium stays in the relatively small interstitial space for a few minutes before exiting through venules or lymphatic vessels [86]. However, in conditions like myocardial infarction, hypertrophic cardiomyopathy (HCM), dilated cardiomyopathy (DCM), and Fabry disease, the collagen matrix of scar tissue increases the interstitial space and myocardial distribution volume of gadolinium, leading to LGE—a marker of myocardial fibrosis. LGE is not specific for fibrosis, as it can also be caused by conditions that significantly increase the interstitial space or slow down gadolinium exit. In some cases of myocarditis, LGE detected within the first week may disappear after 6 months, likely due to interstitial edema or inflammatory cell infiltration [87] [88].

After contrast injection, the gadolinium-based contrast agent concentration varies across different myocardial compartments due to their distinct wash-in and washout kinetics. The presence, location, pattern, and extent of LGE allow for accurate differential diagnosis between ischemic and non-ischemic heart diseases, as well as among various cardiomyopathies [86, 87]. Ischemic LGE patterns always involve the subendocardial layer with varying transmural extent, appearing confluent within a single coronary artery territory [89]. Non-ischemic patterns, however, display mid-wall, subepicardial, or mixed distributions not confined to any coronary territory [86]. As the current cardiac MRI standard for assessing myocardial viability in ischemic cardiomyopathy, LGE can detect even small subendocardial infarcts due to its superior spatial resolution compared to techniques like Single Photon Emission Computed Tomography [90]. Characteristic LGE patterns include patchy/streaky intramyocardial patterns at right ventricular insertion sites in hypertrophic cardiomyopathy, diffuse subendocardial enhancement with early cavity darkening and myocardial nulling in cardiac amyloidosis, midwall or subepicardial basal inferolateral enhancement in Fabry disease, absence of LGE in 75% of dilated cardiomyopathy cases with non-ischemic (20–25%) or ischemic (0–5%) patterns in the remainder, and patchy mid-myocardial or focal subepicardial lesions in cardiac sarcoidosis [86, 87].

The characteristics and extent of LGE on cardiac MRI have significant prognostic implications across various cardiac diseases. In acute myocardial infarction, a meta-analysis by Stone et al. of 2632 patients showed that every 5% increase in infarct size by LGE was associated with 20% higher rates of mortality and heart failure hospitalization [91]. Lee et al. found that LGE extent was a strong predictor of major adverse cardiovascular events over a median 9.4-year follow-up in 146 patients with coronary artery disease undergoing bypass surgery, independent of left ventricular function [92].

Regarding cardiomyopathies, the pattern and distribution of non-ischemic LGE provide prognostic value beyond just its presence. In hypertrophic cardiomyopathy, Chan et al. demonstrated in 1293 patients over a median 3.3-year follow-up that LGE extent ≥15% increases arrhythmic risk [93]. In Fabry disease, Weidemann et al. showed in 32 patients over 3 years that LGE is associated with worse remodeling and arrhythmic outcomes [94]. For dilated cardiomyopathy, Halliday et al. found in 874 patients over 4.9 years that midwall septal LGE, particularly the annular pattern, portends higher arrhythmic risk [95]. LGE also stratifies risk in arrhythmogenic cardiomyopathy, according to Aquaro et al., in 140 patients over 5 years [96]. Beyond cardiomyopathies, LGE provides prognostic data in aortic stenosis, as Weidemann et al. showed in 58 patients over 9 months, its association with worse remodeling after valve intervention [97]. The 2022 ESC cardiomyopathy guidelines now incorporate LGE for phenotypic description, highlighting its clinical relevance [98].

LGE-MRI has become essential for evaluating atrial fibrosis in atrial fibrillation (AF) patients. Extensive pre-ablation atrial fibrosis is associated with lower success rates when catheter ablation targets only pulmonary vein isolation. Therefore, LGE-MRI findings help guide individualized ablation strategies that extend beyond pulmonary vein isolation by identifying the fibrotic substrate that may require additional targeted ablation [99].

While qualitative visual assessment of LGE is often sufficient for most cardiomyopathies, quantitative measurement of LGE extent has shown added prognostic value in ischemic heart disease and hypertrophic cardiomyopathy. Several techniques exist for quantifying LGE, including manual contouring, signal intensity thresholding, multiple standard deviations, full-width half maximum, Otsu auto-thresholding, and Rayleigh curve fitting methods. However, the lack of standardization in LGE quantification across different MRI labs remains a limitation. Moving towards a standardized quantitative approach could enhance the prognostic utility of this powerful cardiac imaging marker, especially in diseases where LGE extent has been shown to provide independent risk prediction. Another key limitation is LGE's reduced capability to detect diffuse myocardial processes, as it relies on comparing enhanced areas to non-enhanced reference myocardium [86, 87].

There are also important considerations with LGE use. Nephrogenic systemic fibrosis is a rare but serious complication of gadolinium contrast agents, although its incidence has decreased substantially in recent years with the use of more stable polycyclic agents. Caution is still warranted in patients with advanced chronic kidney disease (eGFR <30 mL/min/1.73 m2), and dialysis should be scheduled within 12 h of gadolinium administration when no alternative is available [100]. Additionally, interpretation of LGE images should not occur in isolation, but rather in the context of all cardiac MRI sequences, including cine, perfusion, T1/T2 mapping, and other tissue characterization techniques. A comprehensive multiparametric assessment is required for accurate diagnostic evaluation [17]. Recent studies have been using machine learning methods to reduce the utilization of contrast media and obtain similar details as LGE from the non-contrast images [98].

1.4.2 T1, T2, T2* Mapping and ECV Quantification

T1 and T2 mapping are advanced cardiac MRI techniques that quantify myocardial tissue's T1 and T2 relaxation times on a voxel-wise parametric map [101]. Unlike conventional semi-quantitative signal intensity methods, mapping directly quantifies T1, T2, and ECV values. This parametric quantitative approach better evaluates diffuse myocardial processes like myocarditis or fibrosis compared to region-of-interest analyses [102].

T1 (spin-lattice/longitudinal relaxation) maps indicate how quickly nuclei recover equilibrium along the main magnetic field after excitation [103]. T2 (spin-spin/transverse relaxation) maps reflect myocardial water content, with longer T2 times suggesting edema [104]. Both T1 and T2 relaxation times are tissue-specific biomarkers for distinguishing normal and abnormal myocardium [102]. The T1 relaxation time reflects the rate of energy transfer from excited protons to their molecular surroundings, which depends on factors like molecular size, shape, viscosity, temperature, and magnetic field strength. T1 is sensitive to changes in both intracellular and extracellular compartments, being influenced by components such as collagen, proteins, water, lipids, and iron content. Since pathological processes alter the water composition or local molecular environment of tissues, they generally also impact the observed T1 values [102, 103]. Accumulation of edematous fluid leads to increased native T1 relaxation times, a phenomenon more pronounced on T2-weighted sequences. Similarly, fibrotic scar tissue exhibits elevated native T1 values. In contrast, lipid or iron deposition within cells reduces native T1 relaxation times. Pathologies involving edema, inflammation, or infiltrative processes may also manifest as an expansion of the ECV [102, 105].

During cardiac MRI, the death of myocytes leads to an increase in the volume of extracellular fluid in the damaged heart muscle. This causes a delay in the absorption and removal of gadolinium, reducing its T1 relaxation time. As a result, the myocardium appears brighter compared to normal myocardium on T1-weighted inversion-recovery images taken 10–20 min after administering a 0.1–0.2 mmol/kg intravenous dose of gadolinium contrast material on cardiac MR imaging. The LGE images represent the extent of the infarcted myocardium [103, 106]. Currently, only gadobutrol is authorized at a dosage of 0.1 mmol/kg to evaluate myocardial perfusion (stress, rest) and myocardial infarction (LGE imaging).

Additionally, T2* mapping, which quantifies T2* relaxation times, has emerged as a valuable technique for evaluating myocardial iron overload and detecting myocardial hemorrhage. It measures the shortening of T2* relaxation caused by iron deposition [101, 107].

T1 Mapping T1 mapping quantifies the T1 relaxation periods of each myocardial pixel and creates a T1 value map. These maps help patients with diffuse or mild myocardial alterations that cannot be seen on gray-scale imaging [108, 109]. Even isotropic sequences are being designed for 3D mapping [110].

Before late gadolinium enhancement (LGE) sequence changes, pre-contrast T1 mapping can reveal amyloid involvement. Patients with low-flow, low-gradient aortic stenosis and dilated cardiomyopathy have diffuse cardiac fibrosis and high T1 values [111, 112].T1 levels drop in Fabry's disease due to glycosphingolipid buildup [113].

T2 Mapping T2 mapping, like T1 mapping, generates parametric images or maps that describe the relaxation times of the myocardium at type 2 (T2), enabling a possibly more unbiased illustration of inflammation and edema compared to gray-scale T2 imaging. There is increasing evidence that T2 mapping can detect transient inflammation in regions not identified on routine T2 sequences [114]. The current clinical indications for T2 mapping are acute myocarditis, sarcoidosis, inflammation associated with myocardial infarction, toxicity due to chemotherapeutic medications, and cardiac transplant rejection [115–117].

T2* Mapping Heart failure is a prevalent cause of mortality in patients with thalassemia and iron overload. Conventional imaging techniques have limited potential for early detection, as cardiac involvement is only evident after the onset of ventricular dysfunction, which occurs late in the disease's progression. The T2* values facilitate the identification and quantification of iron deposition in the early phases, as well as the monitoring of the treatment response and efficiency of the chelation.

The presence of cardiac iron deposition predicted the adverse prognosis of cardiac iron deposition, and early detection enables the early implementation of chelation in conjunction with other treatment strategies [107]. More recently, T2*mapping has been utilized to identify intramyocardial hemorrhage as an adverse prognosis marker in acute infarction [118].

Extracellular Volume Measurement To measure ECV, native T1 maps are acquired before contrast administration, then co-registered with post-contrast T1 maps obtained after gadolinium injection and equilibration. ECV estimates the extracellular matrix volume fraction using the formula:

$$\mathrm{ECV} = (1 - \mathrm{Hematocrit}) \times \frac{\left(\frac{1}{\mathrm{Post-T1myo}} - \frac{1}{\mathrm{Native-T1myo}}\right)}{\left(\frac{1}{\mathrm{Post-T1Blood}} - \frac{1}{\mathrm{Native-T1Blood}}\right)}.$$

ECV quantifies the myocardial extracellular space and provides a marker of interstitial fibrosis or infiltration. T1/T2 mapping and ECV quantification offer powerful tissue characterization capabilities complementary to late gadolinium enhancement assessment of myocardial fibrosis [101, 119].

These mapping techniques can detect a wide variety of myocardial pathologies: T1 mapping shows increased values in acute coronary syndromes, myocarditis, cardiac sarcoidosis, Takotsubo cardiomyopathy, transplant rejection, amyloidosis, and fibrosis—aiding diagnosis and quantifying tissue changes, while decreased T1 times occur in Anderson-Fabry disease, iron overload, hemorrhage, fatty infiltration, and athlete's heart. T2 mapping highlights myocardial edema in infarction, myocarditis, sarcoidosis, Takotsubo cardiomyopathy, rejection, and amyloidosis, with low T2 associating with iron overload and hemorrhage [101, 119].

In a study by Warnica et al. involving 1876 patients with suspected cardiomyopathy, the incorporation of T1 and T2 mapping in cardiac MRI demonstrated improved diagnostic performance and reader confidence. Specifically, the addition of T1 and T2 mapping enhanced diagnostic sensitivity for myocarditis, Fabry disease, and amyloidosis compared to the core protocol alone. Furthermore, T1 and T2 mapping improved reader diagnostic confidence in 39% of cases evaluated for diagnostic utility [120]. Myocardial mapping techniques like T1, T2, and ECV mapping also enable the detection of subclinical myocardial changes before manifestation on LGE, allowing earlier clinical intervention [102].

Currently, T1, T2, and ECV values are recognized as robust biomarkers for diagnosing cardiomyopathies and as predictive factors for treatment monitoring and prognosis. Several important studies have demonstrated the prognostic value of T1, T2, and ECV mapping in various cardiac conditions. In DCM, a study by Barison et al. assessed 89 DCM patients with a 24-month follow-up. The study found that ECV was independently associated with the occurrence of cardiovascular death, hospitalization for heart failure, and appropriate defibrillator intervention [121]. For HCM, a study by Dass et al. evaluated 28 HCM patients and found that T1 values correlated with disease severity and increased along with increasing wall thickness in HCM [122]. In amyloidosis, Banypersad et al. demonstrated that native T1 values >1044 ms and ECV values >45% were associated with hazard ratios for death of 3.84 and 5.39, respectively [123]. Regarding acute myocardial ischemia, Dall'Armellina et al. assessed 41 ST-elevation myocardial infarction patients and reported a significant relationship between non-contrast T1 mapping and the degree of myocardial damage assessed by LGE or T2-weighted imaging. They noted that T1 values could predict functional recovery after acute myocardial infarction [124]. For patients with transfusion-dependent anemias or hereditary hemochromatosis, severely low myocardial T2* values indicate high cardiac risk. T2* <20 ms signals an increased risk of arrhythmias and systolic dysfunction, while T2* <10 ms indicates a high risk of progressing to overt heart failure [107, 125].

Despite these advances, one major challenge hindering the widespread clinical adoption of T1 and T2 mapping is the variability in native T1 and T2 values due to differences in imaging equipment and sequences. Addressing this issue through the standardization of imaging techniques and developing robust and reproducible mapping protocols is crucial for facilitating the broader clinical application of T1 and T2 mapping in routine practice [126].

1.4.3 Feature Tracking and Strain Analysis

Feature tracking in cardiac MRI is a post-processing technique used to assess myocardial strain, including global longitudinal strain (GLS), global circumferential strain (GCS), and global radial strain (GRS). These parameters quantify myocardial deformation and provide insights into cardiac function beyond ejection fraction. GLS measures the shortening of the myocardium along the heart's long axis, reflecting subendocardial function, often impaired early in diseases like cardiomyopathies. GCS assesses circumferential shortening in short-axis views, indicative of mid-wall myocardial function, and is sensitive to conditions like hypertrophy. GRS evaluates radial thickening from the endocardium to the epicardium and is crucial for detecting changes in ventricular contractility. Feature tracking utilizes standard cine MRI sequences, making it a valuable, non-invasive, and contrast-free tool for evaluating myocardial mechanics in various cardiac conditions [127].

CMR strain imaging is a promising technique for cardiac evaluation that extends beyond conventional functional analysis. It aids in identifying preclinical left ventricular dysfunction prior to overt regional wall motion abnormality and subsequent reduction in ejection fraction by providing information on myocardial deformation. Strain analysis can be conducted by either acquiring specific targeted sequences (CMR labeling) or by employing post-processing techniques to standard cine SSFP sequences, such as feature tracking. CMR tagging is presently recognized as a standard for strain imaging and has been validated [128, 129]. In a prospective investigation that was recently completed, it was demonstrated that left ventricular strain is an independent predictor of adverse cardiac events following vasodilator stress [130]. In addition, feature tracking has demonstrated its potential in the prediction of adverse events in arrhythmogenic cardiomyopathies [131].

Finally, significant progress is being achieved in CMR, namely in the scanning phase and post-processing capabilities. The following section examines technological advancements and progress in cardiac magnetic resonance imaging (CMR), explicitly highlighting enhancements in data acquisition and reconstruction, novel technologies and clinical applications of CMR, MR-guided cardiac procedures, and the contribution of Artificial Intelligence and machine learning in improving the field [132].

Recent advances in CMR data acquisition techniques have significantly improved diagnostic capabilities. These advancements include faster scanning, which reduces the time patients spend in the scanner, and the implementation of respiratory and cardiac gating that enhances image quality by synchronizing with heartbeats and breathing. Whole-heart spatial coverage allows for a comprehensive evaluation of the heart in a single acquisition, while cardiac mapping facilitates detailed visualization of cardiac structures. Stress testing evaluates cardiac function under physical stress, and artifact reduction minimizes distortions for clearer images. Additionally, dimensional (4D) acquisition captures dynamic changes over time, myocardial strain assesses heart muscle deformation, and diffusion-weighted CMR provides insights into tissue characteristics. CMR-guided interventions assist in planning and executing cardiac procedures, and the integration of Artificial Intelligence and machine learning enhances image analysis and interpretation efficiency (Fig. 1.1).

1.4.3.1 Cardiac MRI vs. Other Modalities: Strengths and Weaknesses

Cardiac MRI utilizes powerful magnetic fields and radiofrequency waves to generate highly detailed images of the heart's anatomy, function, and tissue composition [133]. Unlike other modalities, MRI does not use ionizing radiation, making it a safer option for repeated scans, especially in younger patients. Its ability to provide a wealth of information about cardiac structure and function makes it invaluable in diagnosing various heart conditions, from myocardial infarction to congenital heart defects [134].

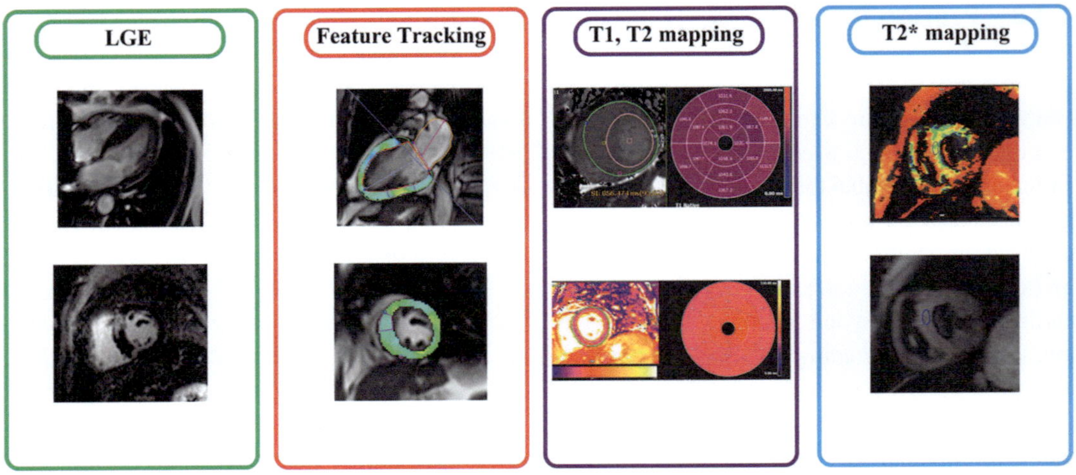

Fig. 1.1 Imaging examples of LGE, feature tracking, T1, T2, and T2* in cardiac magnetic resonance imaging

1.4.3.2 Strengths of Cardiac MRI

- ***High Tissue Contrast and Resolution***: One of the greatest strengths of cardiac MRI is its ability to differentiate between various soft tissues, offering detailed information on myocardial structure, fibrosis, and even blood flow. This makes MRI especially useful for evaluating diseases like cardiomyopathies, myocarditis, and ischemic heart disease [135].
- ***Functional Assessment:*** Cardiac MRI provides dynamic imaging, allowing real-time evaluation of heart function, including ventricular volumes, ejection fraction, and wall motion abnormalities. It is considered the gold standard for measuring these functional parameters [133].
- ***No Ionizing Radiation:*** Unlike CT scans, MRI does not expose patients to radiation, making it suitable for young patients, pregnant women, and those requiring serial imaging over time [136].
- ***Tissue Characterization:*** MRI can assess tissue composition, distinguishing between normal, infarcted, and inflamed myocardium. Techniques such as LGE are essential in identifying myocardial scar tissue, providing important prognostic information in cases like myocardial infarction [137].

1.4.3.3 Weaknesses of Cardiac MRI

- ***Cost and Availability:*** MRI machines are expensive to purchase and maintain. This often makes cardiac MRI less accessible, especially in low-resource settings. Additionally, scans can be time-consuming and require highly specialized personnel for interpretation [138].
- ***Contraindications:*** MRI is not suitable for all patients, particularly those with implanted medical devices like pacemakers or defibrillators, although newer devices may be MRI-compatible [139].
- ***Motion Sensitivity:*** Cardiac MRI is highly sensitive to patient movement and irregular heartbeats, which can reduce image quality. This sometimes necessitates the use of breath-holding techniques or sedatives in certain populations, such as children or claustrophobic patients [140].

Cardiac MRI vs. Computed Tomography (CT)

Cardiac CT, especially coronary CT angiography (CTA), has become a crucial tool for visualizing coronary arteries and calcifications. Unlike MRI, CT scans use X-rays to produce images, making them more accessible and faster, but they expose patients to ionizing radiation [141].

Cardiac CT scans present several key strengths that make them invaluable in clinical practice. They are significantly faster than MRIs, typically completed in just a few minutes, which improves convenience for both patients and clinicians. CT angiography is particularly effective at visualizing coronary arteries and identifying atherosclerotic plaques, playing a crucial role in assessing coronary artery disease. Additionally, the widespread availability of CT scanners in hospitals enhances accessibility to this imaging modality across various healthcare settings, facilitating timely diagnosis and treatment [142].

CT imaging has notable weaknesses, including radiation exposure, which poses risks, particularly with repeated scans, especially in younger patients. While CT excels in providing anatomical details, it is less effective than cardiac MRI in assessing cardiac function, such as wall motion and ejection fraction. Additionally, the use of iodinated contrast agents in CT can lead to allergic reactions and nephropathy, particularly in individuals with kidney disease, whereas MRI utilizes gadolinium-based agents that present a lower risk of nephrotoxicity [143–145].

Cardiac MRI vs. Echocardiography

Echocardiography is the most commonly used imaging modality in cardiology due to its ease of use, real-time imaging capability, and non-invasiveness. It uses ultrasound waves to produce images of the heart, and it is often the first-line tool for evaluating cardiac function and structure [146].

Echocardiography offers several strengths that make it a valuable tool in clinical practice. Its portability and accessibility allow for bedside use, which is particularly beneficial in emergency and outpatient settings. The capability of providing real-time imaging enables effective assessment of valvular function, wall motion, and hemodynamics throughout various phases of the cardiac cycle. Additionally, its lower cost compared to MRI and CT scans enhances its accessibility in routine medical evaluations [147] .

Despite its advantages, echocardiography has notable weaknesses. The resolution of echocardiographic images may be lower than that of MRI or CT, especially in patients with obesity or lung disease, where ultrasound penetration is compromised. Furthermore, the quality of the images is highly dependent on the operator's skill, leading to variability in results across different clinicians. Finally, echocardiography lacks robust tissue characterization capabilities, which limits its effectiveness in identifying myocardial scarring or fibrosis [148].

Each cardiac imaging modality—MRI, CT, and echocardiography—has its unique advantages and drawbacks. While cardiac MRI is unparalleled in tissue characterization and functional assessment without radiation, its high cost and complexity limit its use to specialized settings. CT, on the other hand, excels in rapid anatomical imaging, especially of coronary arteries, but involves radiation exposure. Echocardiography, though more limited in tissue detail, remains the workhorse of cardiac imaging due to its accessibility, real-time imaging, and lower cost. In clinical practice, the choice of modality depends on the specific clinical question, the patient's condition, and the availability of resources.

1.4.3.4 The Future of CMR

The future of CMR imaging is set to advance in two significant areas. First, the evaluation of myocardial tissue characteristics without gadolinium contrast is gaining ground, as emerging research suggests that non-contrast imaging combined with computer analytics can effectively detect fibrosis, matching the efficacy of contrast-enhanced methods [149, 150]. Second, the integration of Artificial Intelligence into CMR promises to revolutionize the field, likely incorporating faster image acquisition and reconstruction algorithms, enhanced diagnostic radiomics, and deep learning models that fuse CMR data with other medical information to improve cardiovascular risk prediction [84]. These developments will be discussed in the upcoming chapters.

References

1. Weiner RB, et al. Blood pressure and left ventricular hypertrophy during American-style football participation. Circulation. 2013;128(5):524–31.
2. O'Donnell R, Armstrong K. The archaeology of 20th-century factory management: four factories on the Team Valley Trading Estate. Ind Archaeol Rev. 2020;42(2):154–69.
3. McGinn S. Progress in the study of cardiovascular disease in 1936. N Engl J Med. 1938;218(18):759–71.
4. Paul O. Background of the prevention of cardiovascular disease. I. Nutritional, infectious, and alcoholic heart disease. Circulation. 1989;79(6):1361–8.
5. de Roos A, Higgins CB. Cardiac radiology: centenary review. Radiology. 2014;273(2 Suppl):S142–59.
6. White PD. Observations on the clinical value of the Roentgen ray in the diagnosis of cardiovascular disease. Am J Roentgenol Radium Ther. 1930;
7. Polevski J. The heart visible. Davis, PA; 1934.
8. Roesler H. Clinical roentgenology of the cardiovascular system. Bailliere; 1937.
9. Hodges FJ. Roentgenological examination of the heart. Radiology. 1926;7(2):116–8.
10. Hodges PC. Estimation of cardiac area in man. Madison: University of Wisconsin—Madison; 1924.
11. Chamberlain WE, Dock W. The study of the heart action with the roentgen cinematograph. Radiology. 1926;7(3):185–9.
12. Eyster JAE. The size of the heart in the normal and in organic heart disease. Radiology. 1927;8(4):300–6.
13. Hodges FJ. The clinical value of roentgen measurements of heart size. Radiology. 1933;20(3):161–4.
14. Rigler LG. The roentgenologic differentiation of lesions of the right and left heart. Radiology. 1933;20(6):463–71.
15. Hirsch IS. The recording of cardiac movements and sounds by the Roentgen ray (kymophonoroentgenography). Radiology. 1934;22(4):403–22.
16. Ungerleider HE, Gubner R. Teleoroentgen Kymography: its application to the study of heart size, output, and aortic elasticity. Radiology. 1939;33(4):497–507.
17. Scott WG, Moore S, McCordock HA. Roentgen kymographic studies of cardiac conditions. Radiology. 1937;28(2):196–210.
18. Robb G, Steinberg I. Visualization of the chambers of the heart, the pulmonary circulation, and the great blood vessels in man-A practical method. Am J Roentgenol Radium Ther. 1939;41:1–17.
19. Castellanos A, et al. On factors intervening in obtention of perfect angiocardiograms. 1938;10:217–23.
20. Grishman A, Steinberg M, Sussman MJR. Tetralogy of Fallot: contrast visualization of heart and great vessels. 1941;37(2):178–80.
21. Paulin, S., Coronary angiography: a technical, anatomic and clinical study. 1964.
22. Taylor HK, Shulman IJR. Cardio-angiography. 1942;39(3):323–33.
23. Abrams HL. An approach to biplane cineangiocardiography. 3. Early clinical observations. Radiology. 1959;73(4):531–8.
24. Abrams HL. An approach to biplane cineangiocardiography.II equipment and procedure. Radiology. 1959;72(5):741–50.
25. Jonsson G, Broden B, Karnell J. Selective angiocardiography. Acta Radiol (Stockh). 1949;32(5–6):486–97.
26. Dotter CT, Frische LH. Visualization of the coronary circulation by occlusion aortography: a practical method. Radiology. 1958;71(4):502–24.
27. Sones FM Jr. Cine coronary arteriography. Mod Concepts Cardiovasc Dis. 1962;31:735–8.
28. Masoomi Z, et al. Prevalence of contrast-induced nephropathy after primary percutaneous coronary intervention at a tertiary referral hospital. Heliyon. 2024;10(4)
29. Webb JA, et al. Late adverse reactions to intravascular iodinated contrast media. Eur Radiol. 2003;13(1):181–4.
30. Gramiak R, Shah PM, Kramer DH. Ultrasound cardiography: contrast studies in anatomy and function. Radiology. 1969;92(5):939–48.
31. Gramiak R, Shah PM. Echocardiography of the normal and diseased aortic valve. Radiology. 1970;96(1):1–8.
32. Biswas M, et al. Two- and three-dimensional speckle tracking echocardiography: clinical applications and future directions. Echocardiography. 2013;30(1):88–105.
33. Muraru D, et al. Three-dimensional speckle-tracking echocardiography: benefits and limitations of integrating myocardial mechanics with three-dimensional imaging. Cardiovasc Diagn Ther. 2018;8(1):101–17.
34. Bonte FJ, et al. A new method for radionuclide imaging of myocardial infarcts. Radiology. 1974;110(2):473–4.
35. Martin ND, et al. Rubidium-81: a new myocardial scanning agent: noninvasive regional myocardial perfusion scans at rest and exercise and comparison with potassium-43. Radiology. 1974;111(3):651–6.
36. Brunken R, et al. PET detection of viable tissue in myocardial segments with persistent defects at T1-201 SPECT. Radiology. 1989;172(1):65–73.
37. Rischpler C, Nekolla S, Schwaiger M. PET and SPECT in heart failure. Curr Cardiol Rep. 2013;15(3):337.
38. Nensa F, et al. Hybrid PET/MR imaging of the heart: feasibility and initial results. Radiology. 2013;268(2):366–73.
39. Lackner K, Thurn P. Computed tomography of the heart: ECG-gated and continuous scans. Radiology. 1981;140(2):413–20.
40. Nasis A, et al. Current and evolving clinical applications of multidetector cardiac CT in assessment of structural heart disease. Radiology. 2013;267(1):11–25.

41. Breen J, et al. Coronary artery calcification detected with ultrafast CT as an indication of coronary artery disease. Radiology. 1992;185(2):435–9.
42. Bielak LF, et al. Small lesions in the heart identified at electron beam CT: calcification or noise? Radiology. 1994;192(3):631–6.
43. Mautner GC, et al. Coronary artery calcification: assessment with electron beam CT and histomorphometric correlation. Radiology. 1994;192(3):619–23.
44. Shaw LJ, et al. Prognostic value of cardiac risk factors and coronary artery calcium screening for all-cause mortality. Radiology. 2003;228(3):826–33.
45. Callister TQ, et al. Coronary artery disease: improved reproducibility of calcium scoring with an electron-beam CT volumetric method. Radiology. 1998;208(3):807–14.
46. Ohnesorge B, et al. Cardiac imaging by means of electrocardiographically gated multisection spiral CT: initial experience. Radiology. 2000;217(2):564–71.
47. Hunold P, et al. Radiation exposure during cardiac CT: effective doses at multi–detector row CT and electron-beam CT. Radiology. 2003;226(1):145–52.
48. Datta J, et al. Anomalous coronary arteries in adults: depiction at multi–detector row CT angiography. Radiology. 2005;235(3):812–8.
49. Schoepf UJ, et al. CT of coronary artery disease. Radiology. 2004;232(1):18–37.
50. Wolf GL, Gerlings ED, Wilson WJ. Depression of myocardial contractility induced by hypertonic coronary injections in the isolated perfused dog heart. Radiology. 1973;107(3):655–8.
51. McNamara MT, et al. Acute myocardial ischemia: magnetic resonance contrast enhancement with gadolinium-DTPA. Radiology. 1984;153(1):157–63.
52. Higgins CB. Early use of contrast in cardiac magnetic resonance. JACC Cardiovasc Imaging. 2009;2(2):241–4.
53. Peters PJ, Reinhardt S. The echocardiographic evaluation of intracardiac masses: a review. J Am Soc Echocardiogr. 2006;19(2):230–40.
54. American College of Cardiology Foundation Appropriate Use Criteria Task, F, et al. ACCF/ASE/AHA/ASNC/HFSA/HRS/SCAI/SCCM/SCCT/SCMR 2011 Appropriate use criteria for echocardiography. A report of the American College of Cardiology Foundation Appropriate Use Criteria Task Force, American Society of Echocardiography, American Heart Association, American Society of Nuclear Cardiology, Heart Failure Society of America, Heart Rhythm Society, Society for Cardiovascular Angiography and Interventions, Society of Critical Care Medicine, Society of Cardiovascular Computed Tomography, and Society for Cardiovascular Magnetic Resonance Endorsed by the American College of Chest Physicians. J Am Coll Cardiol. 2011;57(9):1126–66.
55. den Harder AM, et al. New horizons in cardiac CT. Clin Radiol. 2016;71(8):758–67.
56. O'Donnell DH, et al. Cardiac tumors: optimal cardiac MR sequences and spectrum of imaging appearances. AJR Am J Roentgenol. 2009;193(2):377–87.
57. American College of Cardiology Foundation Task Force on Expert Consensus, D, et al. ACCF/ACR/AHA/NASCI/SCMR 2010 expert consensus document on cardiovascular magnetic resonance: a report of the American College of Cardiology Foundation Task Force on Expert Consensus Documents. J Am Coll Cardiol. 2010;55(23):2614–62.
58. Fathala A, Abouzied M, AlSugair AA. Cardiac and pericardial tumors: a potential application of positron emission tomography-magnetic resonance imaging. World J Cardiol. 2017;9(7):600–8.
59. Giang TH, et al. Detection of coronary artery disease by magnetic resonance myocardial perfusion imaging with various contrast medium doses: first European multi-centre experience. Eur Heart J. 2004;25(18):1657–65.
60. Schwitter J, et al. Assessment of myocardial perfusion in coronary artery disease by magnetic resonance: a comparison with positron emission tomography and coronary angiography. Circulation. 2001;103(18):2230–5.
61. Nagel E, et al. Magnetic resonance perfusion measurements for the noninvasive detection of coronary artery disease. Circulation. 2003;108(4):432–7.
62. Sirajuddin A, et al. Ischemic heart disease: noninvasive imaging techniques and findings. Radiographics. 2021;41(4):990–1021.
63. Herfkens RJ, et al. Nuclear magnetic resonance imaging of the cardiovascular system: normal and pathologic findings. Radiology. 1983;147(3):749–59.
64. Crooks LE, et al. Magnetic resonance imaging strategies for heart studies. Radiology. 1984;153(2):459–65.
65. Fletcher BD, et al. Gated magnetic resonance imaging of congenital cardiac malformations. Radiology. 1984;150(1):137–40.
66. Lanzer P, et al. Cardiac imaging using gated magnetic resonance. Radiology. 1984;150(1):121–7.
67. Stark DD, et al. Magnetic resonance imaging of the pericardium: normal and pathologic findings. Radiology. 1984;150(2):469–74.
68. Masui T, Finck S, Higgins CB. Constrictive pericarditis and restrictive cardiomyopathy: evaluation with MR imaging. Radiology. 1992;182(2):369–73.
69. Amparo EG, et al. Aortic dissection: magnetic resonance imaging. Radiology. 1985;155(2):399–406.
70. Yamada T, Tada S, Harada J. Aortic dissection without intimal rupture: diagnosis with MR imaging and CT. Radiology. 1988;168(2):347–52.
71. Bamberg F, et al. Diabetes mellitus: long-term prognostic value of whole-body MR imaging for the occurrence of cardiac and cerebrovascular events. Radiology. 2013;269(3):730–7.
72. Katz J, et al. Estimation of human myocardial mass with MR imaging. Radiology. 1988;169(2):495–8.

73. Sechtem U, et al. Mitral or aortic regurgitation: quantification of regurgitant volumes with cine MR imaging. Radiology. 1988;167(2):425–30.
74. Atkinson DJ, Edelman RR. Cineangiography of the heart in a single breath hold with a segmented turbo-FLASH sequence. Radiology. 1991;178(2):357–60.
75. Foo TK, et al. Improved ejection fraction and flow velocity estimates with use of view sharing and uniform repetition time excitation with fast cardiac techniques. Radiology. 1995;195(2):471–8.
76. Li D, et al. Coronary arteries: three-dimensional MR imaging with fat saturation and magnetization transfer contrast. Radiology. 1993;187(2):401–6.
77. Duerinckx AJ, Urman MK. Two-dimensional coronary MR angiography: analysis of initial clinical results. Radiology. 1994;193(3):731–8.
78. Wang Y, et al. Navigator-echo-based real-time respiratory gating and triggering for reduction of respiration effects in three-dimensional coronary MR angiography. Radiology. 1996;198(1):55–60.
79. Danias PG, et al. Prospective navigator correction of image position for coronary MR angiography. Radiology. 1997;203(3):733–6.
80. Stuber M, et al. Submillimeter three-dimensional coronary MR angiography with real-time navigator correction: comparison of navigator locations. Radiology. 1999;212(2):579–87.
81. Hundley WG. Fifty years of cardiovascular magnetic resonance: continuing evolution toward the "one-stop shop" for cardiovascular diagnosis. Circulation. 2024;149(24):1859–61.
82. Rabbat MG, et al. The future of cardiac magnetic resonance clinical trials. Washington, DC: American College of Cardiology Foundation; 2022. p. 2127–38.
83. Situ Y, et al. Cardiovascular magnetic resonance imaging for structural heart disease. Cardiovasc Diagn Ther. 2020;10(2):361–75.
84. Morales MA, Manning WJ, Nezafat R. Present and future innovations in AI and cardiac MRI. Radiology. 2024;310(1):e231269.
85. Puntmann VO, et al. Society for Cardiovascular Magnetic Resonance (SCMR) expert consensus for CMR imaging endpoints in clinical research: part I—analytical validation and clinical qualification. J Cardiovasc Magn Reson. 2018;20(1):67.
86. Aquaro GD, et al. Diagnostic and prognostic role of late gadolinium enhancement in cardiomyopathies. Eur Heart J Suppl. 2023;25(Suppl C):C130–6.
87. Holtackers RJ, et al. Late gadolinium enhancement cardiac magnetic resonance imaging: from basic concepts to emerging methods. In: RöFo-Fortschritte auf dem Gebiet der Röntgenstrahlen und der bildgebenden Verfahren. Georg Thieme Verlag KG; 2022.
88. Ghaffari Jolfayi A, et al. Imaging findings in cardiovascular involvements of IgG4-related disease: a systematic review study. Rheumatology. 2024:keae494.
89. McCrohon JA, et al. Differentiation of heart failure related to dilated cardiomyopathy and coronary artery disease using gadolinium-enhanced cardiovascular magnetic resonance. Circulation. 2003;108(1):54–9.
90. West AM, Kramer CM. Cardiovascular magnetic resonance imaging of myocardial infarction, viability, and cardiomyopathies. Curr Probl Cardiol. 2010;35(4):176–220.
91. Stone GW, et al. Relationship between infarct size and outcomes following primary PCI: patient-level analysis from 10 randomized trials. J Am Coll Cardiol. 2016;67(14):1674–83.
92. Lee S-A, et al. Long-term prognostic value of late gadolinium-enhanced magnetic resonance imaging in patients with and without left ventricular dysfunction undergoing coronary artery bypass grafting. Am J Cardiol. 2016;118(11):1647–54.
93. Chan RH, et al. Prognostic value of quantitative contrast-enhanced cardiovascular magnetic resonance for the evaluation of sudden death risk in patients with hypertrophic cardiomyopathy. Circulation. 2014;130(6):484–95.
94. Weidemann F, et al. Long-term effects of enzyme replacement therapy on fabry cardiomyopathy: evidence for a better outcome with early treatment. Circulation. 2009;119(4):524–9.
95. Halliday BP, et al. Outcome in dilated cardiomyopathy related to the extent, location, and pattern of late gadolinium enhancement. JACC Cardiovasc Imaging. 2019;12(8 Pt 2):1645–55.
96. Aquaro GD, et al. Prognostic value of magnetic resonance phenotype in patients with Arrhythmogenic right ventricular cardiomyopathy. J Am Coll Cardiol. 2020;75(22):2753–65.
97. Weidemann F, et al. Impact of myocardial fibrosis in patients with symptomatic severe aortic stenosis. Circulation. 2009;120(7):577–84.
98. Meier C, Eisenblätter M, Gielen S. Myocardial late gadolinium enhancement (LGE) in cardiac magnetic resonance imaging (CMR)—an important risk marker for cardiac disease. J Cardiovasc Dev Dis. 2024;11(2):40.
99. Siebermair J, Kholmovski EG, Marrouche N. Assessment of left atrial fibrosis by late gadolinium enhancement magnetic resonance imaging: methodology and clinical implications. JACC Clin Electrophysiol. 2017;3(8):791–802.
100. Lange S, et al. Nephrogenic systemic fibrosis as a complication after gadolinium-containing contrast agents: a rapid review. Int J Environ Res Public Health. 2021;18(6):3000.
101. Messroghli DR, et al. Clinical recommendations for cardiovascular magnetic resonance mapping of T1, T2, T2* and extracellular volume: a consensus statement by the Society for Cardiovascular Magnetic Resonance (SCMR) endorsed by the European Association for Cardiovascular Imaging (EACVI). J Cardiovasc Magn Reson. 2016;19(1):75.
102. Kim PK, et al. Myocardial T1 and T2 mapping: techniques and clinical applications. Korean J Radiol. 2017;18(1):113–31.

103. Kellman P, Hansen MS. T1-mapping in the heart: accuracy and precision. J Cardiovasc Magn Reson. 2014;16(1):2.
104. O'Brien AT, et al. T2 mapping in myocardial disease: a comprehensive review. J Cardiovasc Magn Reson. 2022;24(1):33.
105. Aquaro GD, et al. Diagnostic role of native T1 mapping compared to conventional magnetic resonance techniques in cardiac disease in a real-life cohort. Diagnostics (Basel). 2023;13(14):2461.
106. Flavian A, et al. Cardiac MRI in the diagnosis of complications of myocardial infarction. Diagn Interv Imaging. 2012;93(7–8):578–85.
107. Triadyaksa P, Oudkerk M, Sijens PE. Cardiac T(2) * mapping: techniques and clinical applications. J Magn Reson Imaging. 2020;52(5):1340–51.
108. Demirkiran A, et al. Cardiovascular magnetic resonance techniques for tissue characterization after acute myocardial injury. European Heart J Cardiovasc Imaging. 2019;20(7):723–34.
109. Taylor AJ, et al. T1 mapping: basic techniques and clinical applications. JACC Cardiovasc Imaging. 2016;9(1):67–81.
110. Qi H, et al. Free-running 3D whole heart myocardial T(1) mapping with isotropic spatial resolution. Magn Reson Med. 2019;82(4):1331–42.
111. Nakamori S, et al. Native T1 mapping and extracellular volume mapping for the assessment of diffuse myocardial fibrosis in dilated cardiomyopathy. JACC Cardiovasc Imaging. 2018;11(1):48–59.
112. Rosa VEE, et al. Myocardial fibrosis in classical low-flow, low-gradient aortic stenosis. Circ Cardiovasc Imaging. 2019;12(5):e008353.
113. Roller FC, et al. Assessment of cardiac involvement in Fabry disease (FD) with native T1 mapping. RoFo. 2019;191(10):932–9.
114. Ferreira VM, et al. Cardiovascular magnetic resonance in nonischemic myocardial inflammation: expert recommendations. J Am Coll Cardiol. 2018;72(24):3158–76.
115. Chaikriangkrai K, et al. Prognostic value of myocardial extracellular volume fraction and T2-mapping in heart transplant patients. JACC Cardiovasc Imaging. 2020;13(7):1521–30.
116. Haslbauer JD, et al. CMR imaging biosignature of cardiac involvement due to cancer-related treatment by T1 and T2 mapping. Int J Cardiol. 2019;275:179–86.
117. Chalian H, et al. The role of cardiac magnetic resonance imaging parameters in prognostication of systemic sclerosis in patients with cardiac involvement: a systematic review of the literature. Acad Radiol. 2024;
118. Carrick D, et al. Myocardial hemorrhage after acute Reperfused ST-segment-elevation myocardial infarction: relation to microvascular obstruction and prognostic significance. Circ Cardiovasc Imaging. 2016;9(1):e004148.
119. Haaf P, et al. Cardiac T1 mapping and extracellular volume (ECV) in clinical practice: a comprehensive review. J Cardiovasc Magn Reson. 2016;18(1):89.
120. Warnica W, et al. Clinical impact of cardiac MRI T1 and T2 parametric mapping in patients with suspected cardiomyopathy. Radiology. 2022;305(2):319–26.
121. Barison A, et al. Prognostic significance of myocardial extracellular volume fraction in nonischaemic dilated cardiomyopathy. J Cardiovasc Med (Hagerstown). 2015;16(10):681–7.
122. Dass S, et al. Myocardial tissue characterization using magnetic resonance noncontrast t1 mapping in hypertrophic and dilated cardiomyopathy. Circ Cardiovasc Imaging. 2012;5(6):726–33.
123. Banypersad SM, et al. T1 mapping and survival in systemic light-chain amyloidosis. Eur Heart J. 2015;36(4):244–51.
124. Dall'Armellina E, et al. Cardiovascular magnetic resonance by non contrast T1-mapping allows assessment of severity of injury in acute myocardial infarction. J Cardiovasc Magn Reson. 2012;14(1):15.
125. Robbers L, et al. The influence of microvascular injury on native T1 and T2* relaxation values after acute myocardial infarction: implications for non-contrast-enhanced infarct assessment. Eur Radiol. 2018;28(2):824–32.
126. Mavrogeni S, et al. T1 and T2 mapping in cardiology: "mapping the obscure object of desire". Cardiology. 2017;138(4):207–17.
127. Pryds K, et al. Myocardial strain assessed by feature tracking cardiac magnetic resonance in patients with a variety of cardiovascular diseases—a comparison with echocardiography. Sci Rep. 2019;9(1):11296.
128. Seetharam K, Lerakis S. Cardiac magnetic resonance imaging: the future is bright. F1000Res. 2019:8.
129. Salmanipour A, et al. The predictive value of cardiac MRI strain parameters in hypertrophic cardiomyopathy patients with preserved left ventricular ejection fraction and a low fibrosis burden: a retrospective cohort study. Front Cardiovasc Med. 2023:10.
130. Romano S, et al. Prognostic implications of blunted feature-tracking global longitudinal strain during vasodilator cardiovascular magnetic resonance stress imaging. JACC Cardiovasc Imaging. 2020;13(1 Pt 1):58–65.
131. MozafaryBazargany M, et al. Value of cardiac magnetic resonance feature-tracking in Arrhythmogenic cardiomyopathy (ACM): a systematic review and meta-analysis. IJC Heart Vasc. 2024;53:101455.
132. Hunter F, Corina I, Mahi LA. Chapter 2: State of the art and new advances: cardiac MRI. In: Denis L, editor. New advances in magnetic resonance imaging. Rijeka: IntechOpen; 2023.
133. Russo V, Lovato L, Ligabue G. Cardiac MRI: technical basis. Radiol Med. 2020;125(11):1040–55.
134. Busse A, et al. Cardiac MRI-update 2020. Radiologe. 2020;60(Suppl 1):33–40.

135. Campbell-Washburn AE, et al. Cardiac MRI at low field strengths. J Magn Reson Imaging. 2024;59(2):412–30.
136. FDA. Benefits and risks [Internet]. U.S. Food and Drug Administration. 2017. Available from https://www.fda.gov/radiation-emitting-products/mri-magnetic-resonance-imaging/benefits-and-risks
137. Karamitsos TD, Arvanitaki A, Karvounis H, Neubauer S, Ferreira VM. Myocardial tissue characterization and fibrosis by imaging. J Cardiovasc Magn Reson. 2019;21(1):1–13. https://doi.org/10.1186/s12968-019-0551-0.
138. Samyn MM, et al. Cost analysis of cardiac MRI for cardiac transplant surveillance. JHLT Open. 6:100136.
139. Barison A, et al. Cardiovascular magnetic resonance: what clinicians should know about safety and contraindications. Int J Cardiol. 2021;331:322–8.
140. Guo R, et al. Emerging techniques in cardiac magnetic resonance imaging. J Magn Reson Imaging. 2022;55(4):1043–59.
141. McCollough CH, et al. Strategies for reducing radiation dose in CT. Radiol Clin North Am. 2009;47(1):27–40.
142. Cademartiri F, et al. Dual-source photon-counting computed tomography—Part I: clinical overview of cardiac CT and coronary CT angiography applications. J Clin Med. 2023;12(11):3627.
143. Kwan AC, et al. Next-generation hardware advances in CT: cardiac applications. Radiology. 2021;298(1):3–17.
144. Al-Sharify ZT, Al-Sharify TA, Al-Sharify NT. A critical review on medical imaging techniques (CT and PET scans) in the medical field. In: IOP conference series: materials science and engineering. IOP Publishing; 2020.
145. McDonald JS, et al. Prevention of allergic-like reactions at repeat CT: steroid pretreatment versus contrast material substitution. Radiology. 2021;301(1):133–40.
146. Otto CM. Textbook of clinical echocardiography. Elsevier Health Sciences; 2013.
147. Keller M, et al. Echocardiography as a tool to assess cardiac function in critical care-a review. Diagnostics (Basel). 2023;13(5)
148. Mantella LE, Liblik K, Johri AM. Vascular imaging of atherosclerosis: strengths and weaknesses. Atherosclerosis. 2021;319:42–50.
149. Dastidar AG, et al. Native T1 mapping to detect extent of acute and chronic myocardial infarction: comparison with late gadolinium enhancement technique. Int J Cardiovasc Imaging. 2019;35(3):517–27.
150. Mohammadzadeh A, et al. Native T1, T2 mapping and strain analysis to assess myocardial viability in the subacute phase of MI: comparison with late gadolinium enhancement; 2023. https://doi.org/10.21203/rs.3.rs-2821311/v1.

Deep Learning and Convolutional Neural Networks in Image Processing: Focusing on Cardiac MRI Analysis

2

Amir Ghaffari Jolfayi, Amirhossein Poopak, Reza Elahi, Mohammadhossein Mozafarybazargany, Amir Azimi, and Seyed Amir Ahmad Safavi-Naini

Abstract

Artificial Intelligence (AI), with a focus on machine learning (ML) and deep learning (DL), has become a cornerstone in the advancement of cardiac MRI analysis. This article explores the integration of supervised, unsupervised, and semi-supervised learning approaches, highlighting their distinct roles in addressing challenges like data annotation and achieving high diagnostic accuracy. Supervised learning methods excel in image segmentation and classification tasks, leveraging labeled datasets to detect structural and functional abnormalities. In contrast, unsupervised and semi-supervised paradigms uncover patterns in raw datasets and reduce the reliance on extensive manual labeling.

Central to this discussion is the application of convolutional neural networks (CNNs) in cardiac MRI, enabling automated segmentation, disease classification, and functional parameter estimation. Architectural advancements such as U-Net models, attention mechanisms, and transfer learning are examined, demonstrating their potential to enhance model accuracy and efficiency while addressing challenges like dataset variability and imbalances. Data preprocessing techniques, including normalization, augmentation, and reconstruction, are presented as essential strategies for improving image quality and model generalizability.

The present chapter also addresses key ethical and regulatory considerations, advocating for explainable AI and federated learning to ensure transparency, trust, and compliance in clinical applications. Emerging trends, such as 4D modeling, multimodal data integration, and real-time analysis, are discussed, showcasing the potential for further innovation in cardiac imaging.

This comprehensive analysis underscores the transformative role of AI in cardiology, offering tools to improve diagnostic precision, streamline workflows, and enhance patient outcomes. By combining advanced computa-

Authors Amir Ghaffari Jolfayi, Amirhossein Poopak and Amir Azimi have contributed equality and shared the first co-authorship.

A. Ghaffari Jolfayi · A. Poopak
M. Mozafarybazargany · A. Azimi
Cardiovascular Imaging Research Center, Rajaie Cardiovascular Institute, Tehran, Iran

R. Elahi
Department of Radiology, Zanjan University of Medical Sciences, Zanjan, Iran

S. A. A. Safavi-Naini (✉)
Division of Data-Driven and Digital Medicine (D3M), Icahn School of Medicine at Mount Sinai, New York, NY, USA

A. Ghaffari Jolfayi (ed.), *Navigating Cardiology's Future*,
https://doi.org/10.1007/978-981-95-0313-1_2

tional techniques with clinical expertise, the adoption of AI-driven solutions in cardiac MRI holds the promise of a more efficient and accurate healthcare future.

Keywords

Cardiac magnetic resonance imaging · Deep learning · Machine learning · Artificial intelligence · Convolutional neural network · Image processing

Understanding the Basics of Artificial Intelligence

"Machine intelligence is the last invention that humanity will ever need to make."

Nick Bostrom

2.1 Introduction

Artificial Intelligence (AI) is a rapidly advancing field focused on developing computer systems that can recognize patterns in data and assist humans in complex problem-solving. Since its beginnings in the 1950s, AI has grown from basic rule-based programs to an extensive array of methods capable of aiding disease diagnosis and solving difficult tasks. Groundbreaking contributions from early researchers, such as Christopher Strachey—who developed one of the first AI programs in 1951—and John McCarthy—who introduced the term "Artificial Intelligence" at the 1956 Dartmouth Conference—paved the way for modern AI [1, 2]. Today, AI encompasses a diverse set of techniques, including machine learning (ML), deep learning (DL), and natural language processing (NLP), all designed to augment human intelligence rather than replace it [1, 3].

2.1.1 Machine Learning (ML)

ML is a core component of AI, enabling computer systems to learn and improve from data without relying solely on explicit programming. By identifying patterns in datasets, ML tools support humans in making evidence-based decisions. ML methods can be broadly categorized into various approaches [4–7]:

- Supervised learning: Algorithms are trained on labeled data that map inputs to known outputs. Techniques such as linear/logistic regression, decision trees, and survival analysis build predictive models that help classify or forecast new observations.
- Unsupervised learning: These methods uncover inherent structures or patterns in unlabeled data. Common techniques include clustering algorithms, principal component analysis, and self-organizing maps, each revealing hidden relationships within the dataset.
- Reinforcement learning: This approach focuses on trial-and-error learning within dynamic environments. An agent learns by taking actions, receiving rewards or penalties, and refining its behavior to maximize long-term outcomes [4–7].

In all these scenarios, human expertise and guidance remains central, guiding the choice of algorithms, interpreting results, and validating whether findings align with clinical or research objectives.

2.1.2 Deep Learning (DL)

DL, a specialized subset of ML, draws inspiration from the structure and function of the human brain's neural networks. It employs multi-layered artificial neural networks to extract complex features from large volumes of raw data. Building upon the foundational work of Walter Pitts and Warren McCulloch in 1944, DL has driven breakthroughs in computer vision, language processing, and predictive analytics. Several types of DL networks each serve a unique purpose:

I. Convolutional Neural Networks (CNNs): Widely used for image-based tasks such as classification, object detection, and segmentation, including applications in cardiac MRI analysis [4].

II. Recurrent Neural Networks (RNNs) like LSTMs and GRUs are designed for sequential data like text and speech. Autoencoders are unsupervised networks that learn efficient coding of input data for dimensionality reduction and data generation.
III. Generative Adversarial Networks (GANs) consist of two competing networks that generate highly realistic synthetic data samples. Deep Belief Networks (DBNs) are probabilistic generative models of multiple layers of latent variables [7–9].

2.1.3 Natural Language Processing: Understanding Human Language

NLP enables computers to comprehend, interpret, and generate human language. This domain is crucial in healthcare for tasks such as text classification, information extraction, and the development of chatbot interfaces. When combined with ML, NLP helps distill vast amounts of unstructured information—such as electronic health records—into actionable insights for improved clinical decision support, enhanced diagnostic tools, and faster knowledge discovery in medical research [4, 10].

Figure 2.1 illustrates how AI, ML, DL, and NLP interrelate to form a cohesive ecosystem that supports human intelligence.

2.1.4 AI Development Pipeline

Implementing a comprehensive and effective workflow for ML and AI is crucial for successful clinical deployment. This process requires a rigorous approach from problem formulation to model design, rigorous validation, and continuous refinement. Here, we outline the workflow to guide professionals through the complex process of developing, deploying, and maintaining ML models [4, 11]. The key steps include:

I. Problem Identification: Clearly define the clinical or research question to ensure alignment with real-world needs and current workflows.
II. Data Collection and Management: Gather data from diverse sources—such as imaging systems and electronic health records—while maintaining rigorous storage and quality-control measures. Preprocessing involves managing missing values, removing irrelevant information, and preserving data integrity.
III. Data Exploration and Preprocessing: Analyze data distributions and relationships using statistical methods and visualizations. Use feature engineering and transformations (e.g., normalization, scaling, encoding) to prepare high-quality inputs for modeling.
IV. Model Selection: Choose an appropriate model (e.g., supervised, unsupervised, or

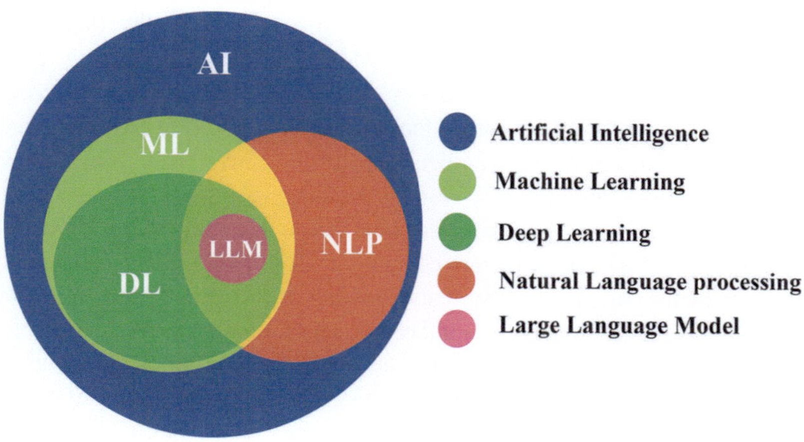

Fig. 2.1 Hierarchical relationships among Artificial Intelligence (AI), Machine Learning (ML), Deep Learning (DL), Natural Language Processing (NLP), and Large Language Models (LLMs)

reinforcement learning) based on the type of data, clinical goals, and performance requirements.

V. Training, Validation, and Testing: Partition the dataset into training, validation, and testing subsets.
   - *Training Set*: Optimize model parameters to minimize the chosen objective function.
   - *Validation Set*: Evaluate and tune hyperparameters, monitoring bias and variance with metrics like accuracy, area under the ROC curve, or the Dice coefficient.
   - *Testing Set*: Confirm the final model's generalization ability on unseen data.
   - Hyperparameter tuning often leverages techniques like cross-validation to reduce overfitting and better estimate real-world performance. Once the model performs well on the validation set, test it on the hold-out data to confirm its generalization ability.

VI. Deployment and Continuous Refinement: Deploy the validated model in a clinical setting and monitor its performance as new data becomes available. Periodically retrain and update the model with additional samples to maintain accuracy and adapt to evolving clinical demands. This iterative cycle of problem definition, model development, validation, and refinement ensures the creation of robust, well-generalizing AI solutions.

2.1.5 Big Data in Healthcare

The healthcare industry produces massive amounts of information, leading to the generation of big data from sources such as electronic health records (EHRs), medical test results, imaging records, clinical notes, and inpatient interviews. This healthcare data is characterized by high volume, velocity, variety, and veracity, making it highly challenging to manage and analyze using traditional methods. As Pat Gelsinger said, "Data is the new science. Big Data holds the answers." While big data has become invaluable for providing additional clinical insights, improving patient care, and aiding clinical guidelines, many valuable findings may remain unrecognized due to the immense scope of captured information. However, AI techniques can have a profound impact by effectively analyzing and deciphering key relationships and insights hidden within the vast troves of healthcare big data, unlocking the answers held within [4, 12, 13].

2.2 Role of AI in Cardiology

Cardiology has embraced AI as a powerful tool to enhance diagnostic accuracy, treatment planning, and patient care. AI techniques have been applied in various areas of cardiology, including:

2.2.1 Cardiovascular Imaging

AI, particularly DL techniques, revolutionizes cardiovascular imaging by providing automated, quantitative, and consistent analysis across all major imaging modalities. In echocardiography, AI algorithms can automatically identify imaging views and cardiac cycles, segment cardiac chambers, quantify volumes and function, detect wall motion abnormalities, and even differentiate between diseases with similar appearances. This reduces operator variability and subjectivity in interpretation. AI also enhances image quality through denoising and artifact removal [3, 14–17]. AI improves image quality for cardiac computed tomography (CT), enables accurate coronary calcium scoring and comprehensive plaque characterization, including stenosis grading, and can estimate fractional flow reserve noninvasively from CT angiography data-matching invasive measurements [14, 18, 19]. DL models used with cardiac MRI have accelerated scan times, provided precise automated segmentation and quantification of structural metrics like volumes and mass, and allowed assessment of function and scar burden [14, 20, 21]. The impact of AI spans nuclear imaging techniques as well. For myocardial perfusion imaging with SPECT or PET, ML models aid in detecting perfusion defects, localizing ischemia, and predicting which patients would benefit from early revascularization based on the imaging findings [22, 23].

2.2.2 Electrocardiogram (ECG) Analysis

AI and ML models have shown impressive capabilities in automated ECG interpretation, often outperforming human experts in detecting conditions like long QT syndrome, atrial fibrillation, and ST-segment abnormalities. These AI-powered ECG algorithms can accurately distinguish normal from abnormal ECGs and confidently diagnose arrhythmias like atrial fibrillation, ventricular tachycardia, and myocardial infarction. AI can empower primary care physicians and non-cardiologists with reasonable sensitivity and specificity to make prompt decisions regarding specialized cardiac care needs. AI-based ECG analysis finds applications in monitoring heart rate variability routine arrhythmia detection in wearable devices [24, 25].

2.2.3 Risk Stratification and Preventive Cardiology

One of the promising areas where AI demonstrates significant potential is preventive cardiology, wherein ML models can be utilized for risk stratification. This data-driven approach can identify patients at high risk of cardiovascular complications, thereby enhancing preventive efforts. As ML algorithms can incorporate numerous variables without preselecting important ones or making prior assumptions, they are well-suited for developing clinical risk prediction models. ML models can integrate traditional and non-traditional risk factors for effective risk stratification. Various ML techniques, such as naive Bayes, k-nearest neighbors, decision trees, random forests, and XGBoost, have been previously employed for predicting adverse cardiac events following ST-elevation myocardial infarction (STEMI) [22, 25].

Finally, the application of AI in cardiovascular imaging is an emerging area with significant promise to enhance diagnostic capabilities and serve as a valuable prognostic tool due to its remarkable capacity to analyze vast amounts of data. However, it is crucial to approach the integration of AI with prudence, viewing these algorithms as complementary aids to augment, rather than substitute, the specialized knowledge and expertise of medical professionals. As we look ahead, the prospects of incorporating AI into patient care are promising and exciting, indicating that the future impact of this transformative technology is already unfolding [26].

2.3 Supervised, Unsupervised, and Semi-supervised Approaches in Cardiac MRI Analysis

ML has become a pivotal tool in modern healthcare, especially in medical image analysis. A clear grasp of supervised and unsupervised learning principles is essential for professionals and researchers aiming to apply ML models effectively in cardiac MRI. While supervised learning relies on labeled data to make predictions, unsupervised learning uncovers intrinsic structures in unlabeled datasets. Additionally, semi-supervised methods merge aspects of both, and reinforcement learning leverages rewards for iterative learning [27, 28]. There are also other types of ML, including reinforcement learning (which performs closely to human psychology by utilizing a reward function) and semi-supervised learning (which involves features of both supervised and unsupervised learning). This section contrasts supervised and unsupervised methods and highlights their key applications in cardiac MRI (CMR) analysis.

2.3.1 Supervised Learning

Supervised models train on labeled data for tasks like diagnosis, classification, outcome prediction, and regression. An expert must label or annotate the dataset beforehand (e.g., normal vs. pathological CMR images). This iterative training process refines predictive accuracy on unseen data. In CMR analysis, supervised models can detect structural or functional abnormalities by mapping labeled inputs (MRI images) to outputs (labels). For instance, cardiologists often label CMR images for segmentation, enabling models—particularly CNNs—to learn automated segmentation of key cardiac structures [29].

Despite this, supervised learning has a significant limitation: reliance on labeled data. Most medical data is raw and unlabeled, and manual labeling of these datasets requires substantial resources, time, and expertise, making the process labor-intensive and costly [30, 31]. Supervised models are typically employed for regression tasks (e.g., identifying relationships between dependent and independent variables) and classification tasks (e.g., categorizing images into predefined classes, such as binary or multiclass classification). Common models include logistic regression and decision trees, random forests, k-nearest neighbors (KNN), and Naive Bayes for classification [28].

2.3.2 Unsupervised Learning

Unsupervised learning, on the other hand, trains models on raw, unlabeled datasets. In unsupervised learning, the goal is to discover data patterns and relationships without the supervisor's guidance. These models autonomously discover similarities and differences in patterns, structures, and relationships within the data without human intervention [28]. Unsupervised learning models typically require large datasets to effectively identify meaningful patterns and clusters. Although human input may be necessary to set certain hyperparameters (e.g., the number of clusters), the model processes large volumes of data with minimal supervision. These models are useful for revealing hidden relationships, trends, and anomalies, making them valuable and appropriate tools for exploratory data analysis [28].

Unsupervised learning is mostly applied to clustering tasks, where data points are grouped based on similarities or to identify associations between variables. This approach is beneficial in the initial stages of data analysis, helping researchers uncover previously unknown structures and relationships in the data, which can guide further investigation. Another application of unsupervised learning is to find an association to discover rules that describe large portions of your data [32]. Examples of unsupervised learning algorithms are K-means clustering, Principal Component Analysis (PCA), Independent Component Analysis (ICA), Autoencoders (AEs), Restricted Boltzmann Machines (RBMs), Deep Belief Networks (DBNs), GANs, and Hierarchical clustering [33]. Table 2.1 describes the main differences between unsupervised and supervised learning models in image analysis.

2.3.3 Semi-supervised (Self-Supervised) Learning

Semi-supervised and self-supervised learning approaches combine elements of both supervised and unsupervised paradigms, enabling models to learn from a large pool of unlabeled samples alongside a comparatively small set of labeled data. In cardiac MRI, where collecting well-annotated images is both time- and resource-intensive, semi-supervised strategies can substantially reduce the annotation burden. By leveraging features learned from unlabeled scans, these models can effectively capture structural and textural information relevant to the heart, thus improving performance on downstream tasks (e.g., classification, segmentation) even when labeled examples are limited. Recent advances in self-supervised learning—such as contrastive learning and masked-image modeling—further enhance feature extraction by pretraining models on unlabeled data. Subsequently, a refined, task-specific training step on fewer labeled samples can deliver accurate diagnostic tools with lower reliance on extensive manual labeling [34, 35].

Table 2.1 Main differences between unsupervised, semisupervised, and supervised learning models in image analysis

Features	Supervised learning	Semisupervised learning	Unsupervised learning
Need for labeled data	Yes	Requires a small amount of labeled data combined with a large amount of unlabeled data	No
Definition of output before training	Yes	Partially defined; uses both labeled and unlabeled data to improve predictions	No
Human supervision	Required	Minimal; limited to providing the labeled subset	Not required
Accuracy	More accurate	Balance of both; accuracy depends on the ratio of labeled to unlabeled data and the algorithm used	Less accurate
Model's complexity	Less complex	Medium complexity; uses methods that blend supervised and unsupervised approaches	More complex
Common algorithms	Support vector machine, deep neural network, k-nearest neighbor, logistic regression, linear regression, decision tree, random forest	Semi-supervised SVM, self-training, label propagation, deep semi-supervised Learning (e.g., consistency regularization methods)	Hierarchical clustering, K-means clustering, autoencoders (AEs), generative adversarial networks (GANs), deep belief networks (DBNs), support vector machine, restricted Boltzmann machines (RBMs)
Number of classes	Usually defined before training	Partially defined; learns from both defined and undefined classes	Usually not defined before training

2.3.4 Applications of Supervised ML Models in Cardiac MRI Analysis

Supervised models are a favorite method in medical imaging since the final goal is to develop models with similar performance to human experts. In recent years, ML models have significantly transformed CMR image analysis. Specific applications include diagnosis, classification, risk stratification, and outcome prediction for various pathologies, such as quantifying myocardial perfusion in coronary artery disease (CAD), classifying myocardial fibrotic tissue, diagnosing ventricular anomalies, and detecting valve abnormalities. Among these, supervised ML models are particularly prevalent in CMR analysis due to their ability to closely replicate the performance of cardiologists [36].

Supervised ML models require labeled data for training. For instance, when training a model for image segmentation, appropriate high-quality segmentation is commonly conducted manually by an expert to define the contours of the myocardium and cardiac chambers to create ground-truth data. The manual segmentation process is time-consuming and depends on the expert's experience. DL models, such as convolutional neural networks, can be applied to provide highly accurate and automated CMR segmentation. These segmented images are then used to train the model to segment subsequent images accurately [37–39]. In a study, Winther and colleagues [40] employed a DL network to automatically segment the epicardium, endocardium, left and right ventricles. The network assessed cardiac function parameters and volumes from various multi-center datasets. Compared to human experts, their DL model achieved a comparable outcome. Similarly, Tan et al. (2017) [41] evaluated the function of a supervised CNN to segment LV automatically in all short-axis slices.

They employed their model on several publicly available datasets. Their model achieved a 0.77 Jaccard index for the LV segmentation challenge dataset.

CMR image acquisition is often challenging since its quality is commonly affected by cardiac and respiratory motion artifacts. Possible solutions for the acceleration of CMR image acquisition are real-time imaging, compressed sensing (CS), and parallel imaging [42, 43]. In addition to segmentation, supervised ML models have been extensively applied to reconstruct CMR images. Traditionally, acquiring high-quality CMR images necessitates skilled operators with precise attention during manual image acquisition. However, ML models can potentially automate or significantly expedite this process. Recent advancements have concentrated on automating tasks such as image acquisition plane planning, heart localization, frequency optimization, and detecting and correcting CMR artifacts [44–46]. DL models have several advantages, including high efficacy, fast reconstruction speed, and higher quality. These features have made DL models more clinically applicable for CMR reconstruction [37].

It is postulated that medical images, including CMR, contain far more information than can be perceived by the human eye alone. Quantitative computational techniques, such as radiomics, enable the extraction of this hidden information. Radiomics, a recently developed quantitative method, facilitates extracting high-throughput hand-crafted features from medical images [31, 47]. ML models extract texture, contrast, and wavelet features from CMR images and leverage them to perform classification or regression tasks. Supervised ML models based on radiomics have been extensively investigated for their potential in diagnosing, classifying, and predicting the prognosis of various cardiac pathologies, including hypertrophic cardiomyopathy (HCM) [48, 49], myocardial fibrosis, myocarditis, myocardial infarction (MI) [50–53], myocarditis [54], and post-MI arrhythmia [55].

In a study, Zhang et al. (2019) [56] employed a three-stage DL pipeline to diagnose chronic MI on a dataset of 212 patients with nonenhanced MRI and 87 healthy control patients. Their model achieved excellent performance in diagnosing chronic MI, with a sensitivity of 90% and specificity of 99%. Kotu et al. (2015) [55] applied supervised ML to predict arrhythmia following MI. Their study demonstrated that the combination of CMR-derived texture features and scar size/location on CMR effectively stratified patient risk, yielding results comparable to established criteria such as scar size and left ventricular ejection fraction (LVEF).

Neisius et al. (2019) [57] utilized radiomic features from T1 CMR to differentiate hypertensive heart disease and HCM. Their support vector machine (SVM) model achieved 80.0% accuracy on the validation set and 86.2% on the training set, surpassing the performance of native T1 mapping. In another study, Baessler et al. (2018) employed a texture feature model based on 1.5 T T2 and T1 maps from 39 subjects to diagnose acute infarct-like myocarditis. The combination of T2 run-length non-uniformity and grey-level non-uniformity texture features resulted in an AUC of 0.88, with a specificity of 92% and a sensitivity of 89%, outperforming the commonly used Lake Louise criteria (LLC) [54].

ML models have also distinguished between viable and non-viable cardiac fibrotic tissues. Larroza et al. (2018) [50] developed a texture-based model to differentiate between viable, non-viable, and remote infarcted segments on cine MRI from 50 patients with chronic MI. Their model demonstrated an AUC of 0.849, with a sensitivity of 85% for detecting remote segments, 72% for viable segments, and 92% for non-viable segments. In another study, Fahmy et al. [58] used a supervised fully convolutional neural network (FCN) for CMR native T1 mapping. Their model enabled the measurement of diffuse myocardial fibrotic tissue. They introduced the FCN model could automatically measure regional and global myocardial T1 values similar to manual measurements by experts.

Pulmonary artery hypertension (PAH) diagnosis is a manual process that needs to be conducted by an expert cardiologist. However, ML models can be employed to diagnose PAH automatically. For example, Swift et al. applied an ML network to diagnose PAH in CMR automatically. Their model showed an AUC of 0.92 for PAH diagnosis, which was less time-consuming and was also superior to the CMR metrics ($p < 0.001$) [59].

In terms of prognosis prediction, supervised ML models have shown significant promise in forecasting adverse cardiovascular events. Venkatesh et al. applied a random survival forest model to predict cardiovascular events in patients with atherosclerosis. Their findings revealed that the random survival forest model outperformed traditional risk scores, with a reduction in the Brier score by 10%–25%. Among the various risk factors, Troponin-T and left ventricular function and structure were the most critical predictors of incident heart failure. Furthermore, the Coronary Artery Calcium (CAC) score was found to be an accurate predictor of all atherosclerotic cardiovascular diseases and coronary heart disease [60].

Finally, effective supervised learning model performance requires large, well-labeled datasets. Generally, the larger the labeled dataset, the better the model's predictive accuracy in supervised learning tasks will be.

2.3.5 Applications of Unsupervised ML Models in Cardiac MRI Analysis

In unsupervised analysis of CMR images, data is introduced to the model without prior annotation or labeling. For instance, a dataset containing both pathological and normal images can be provided. Then, the model learns the inherent characteristics of the images to classify them as normal or pathological. The application of unsupervised models is limited in medical imaging [61].

While unsupervised learning models are less effective for predictive tasks, they excel in uncovering hidden relationships and structures within the data. This makes them valuable for exploratory analysis rather than for building predictive models. A notable example is the study by Oksuz et al. (2018) [44], which employed an unsupervised, fully automated dictionary learning method to jointly analyze motion and appearance for 2D segmentation of the myocardium using a CINE Blood-Oxygen-Level-Dependent (BOLD) CMR dataset. Their model outperformed state-of-the-art supervised segmentation techniques, achieving a 10% higher Dice score (DSC).

Thus, unsupervised learning is particularly useful for identifying patterns and relationships that may not be readily apparent through supervised methods. For example, Verzosa et al. [62] applied an unsupervised topological data analysis (TDA) model to identify phenotypic presentations of LV response in patients with aortic stenosis (AS). Their study demonstrated that multi-feature evaluation using unsupervised ML could accurately recognize LV response patterns as AS progresses.

Some unsupervised methods have been used to learn features from unlabeled CMR data that can later be used in downstream tasks such as classification or disease prediction. For example, Mukhopadhyay et al. (2020) [63] used an unsupervised DL to extract features from CMR images. They combined the model with other clinical data to enhance the diagnostic power of supervised classification models.

According to published studies, supervised ML and DL models have shown great potential for risk stratification, classification, diagnosis, and prognosis prediction of different cardiovascular abnormalities. Nevertheless, unsupervised learning has been less used and still holds great potential for application in cardiovascular imaging.

2.4 Convolutional Neural Networks in CMR

CNNs have revolutionized the image recognition field. Their capacity to learn hierarchical, feature-rich representations directly from raw data makes them a powerful tool with many applications. While CNNs originated in natural image processing, where they excel in tasks such as object detection, facial recognition, and image classification, they have found a particularly impactful role in medical imaging.

Ultrasound, CT, and MRI scans often consist of complex, high-dimensional data that can be hard to process, even for expert physicians. CNNs privileged the advantage of learning to automatically extract relevant and insightful features from these complex images, reducing the extensive engineering features [64]. In recent years, CNN-based techniques have demonstrated state-of-the-art performance in tackling diverse medical imaging tasks, ranging from segmentation and classification to the more complex functions of estimation of the disease prognosis of the patient [65, 66].

Cardiac MRI is one of the most precise imaging modalities in cardiology. It provides detailed structural and functional information about the heart and its surrounding vasculature. A cardiac MRI reveals the health of heart muscle tissue, identifies scarring, assesses perfusion, and measures important parameters such as ejection fraction and cardiac output. However, these images can be challenging to interpret due to their high dimensionality and subtle variations in tissue properties. Additionally, the heart's structures and dimensions vary from patient to patient, and different diseases can manifest differently within MRI data. This is exactly where CNNs have shown great promise. By learning filters that detect features at multiple levels of abstraction, CNNs can identify subtle structural and functional patterns that may improve the diagnosis or monitoring of cardiac pathologies [67].

The following will explore the fundamental concepts of CNN architecture, the unique challenges posed by cardiac imaging, techniques for improving model performance, and the future outlook of CNNs in cardiac MRI analysis.

2.4.1 Overview of CNNs in Image Recognition

CNNs draw inspiration from the visual cortex in animals [68]. They employ a mathematical operation called convolution, which involves sliding small filters (also called kernels) across the image. These filters effectively scan for particular features—such as edges, corners, or more complex textures—by computing dot products between the filter values and the underlying local region in the image [69]. This process of convolving filters over the image allows CNNs to capture local dependencies in a hierarchical manner (Fig. 2.2 and Table 2.2).

I. ***Convolutional Layers:*** The convolutional layers are the primary building blocks of a CNN. Early convolutional layers tend to learn low-level features, such as edges and simple textures. As data flows deeper into the network, these features become more complex and representative of higher-level concepts (e.g., specific anatomical shapes in the case of medical images) [70].
II. ***Pooling Layers:*** Pooling layers (commonly max or average pooling) follow convolutional layers to reduce the spatial dimensions of the feature maps. By summarizing local regions into a single value, pooling helps the network become more robust to small shifts, rotations, and distortions in the input image [71].
III. ***Fully Connected Layers:*** Toward the end of a classic CNN architecture, one or more fully connected layers integrate the spatially reduced features into a global vector that can be used for classification or regression. However, in many modern architectures, fully connected layers are often replaced or complemented by global pooling or specialized layers to handle specific tasks (e.g., segmentation, detection) [72].
IV. ***Activation Functions:*** Non-linear activation functions like ReLU (Rectified Linear Unit), Sigmoid, or Tanh are used after each convolution or fully connected operation. These activations enable the network to learn complex, non-linear mappings between images and target outputs [73].
V. ***Regularization Techniques:*** CNNs can have millions of parameters and are prone to overfitting. Techniques like dropout, data augmentation, and weight decay help prevent overfitting. These regularization strategies are fundamental for medical imaging data, where obtaining large labeled datasets can be difficult [74].

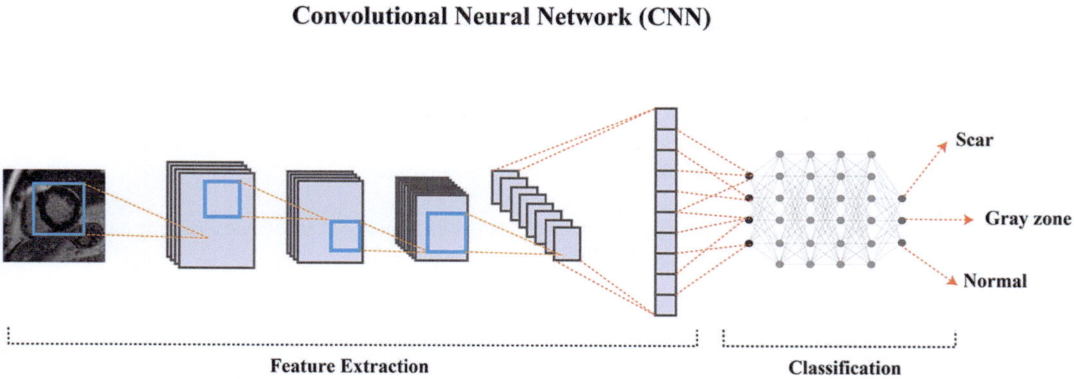

Fig. 2.2 The architecture of a routine Convolutional Neural Network in image processing

Table 2.2 Overview of CNNs and their applications in cardiac MRI analysis

Section	Subsection	Description
A) Overview of CNNs in image recognition	Convolutional layers	Use convolutions to learn low-level (e.g., edges) to high-level features (e.g., anatomical shapes)
	Pooling layers	Reduce spatial dimensions via max or average pooling, improving robustness to shifts and distortions
	Fully connected layers	Combine features for classification or regression; often replaced with global pooling in modern architectures
	Activation functions	Non-linear functions (e.g., ReLU, sigmoid) enable learning of complex mappings between inputs and outputs
	Regularization techniques	Methods like dropout, data augmentation, and weight decay prevent overfitting. Essential for limited medical datasets
B) Applying CNNs to cardiac MRI	Segmentation of cardiac structures	Segment heart structures for accurate clinical measurements (e.g., ejection fraction). U-net architectures excel in this task
	Automated diagnosis	Classify cardiac conditions (e.g., hypertrophic cardiomyopathy) based on MRI features
	Functional parameter estimation	Compute functional metrics (e.g., stroke volume) by tracking cardiac motion through frames
	Feature extraction for prognostic modeling	Use CNN-extracted features for risk stratification and survival analysis
C) Challenges in CNN-based cardiac MRI analysis	Limited and imbalanced datasets	Small datasets and rare conditions create challenges; mitigated with augmentation, synthetic data, and transfer learning
	Variability in image acquisition	Differences in protocols and scanners require normalization and domain adaptation for robustness
	Temporal component	Cardiac motion analysis demands 3D or 4D modeling, increasing computational requirements
	Explainability and trust	Techniques like saliency maps aid in understanding model decisions, essential for clinical adoption
	Regulatory and ethical considerations	Models must meet stringent clinical validation and address privacy and bias concerns

(continued)

Table 2.2 (continued)

Section	Subsection	Description
D) Techniques and advances for improved CNN performance	U-net and variants	U-net and its variants (e.g., attention U-net) are widely used for segmentation tasks
	Multi-view and multi-task learning	Leverage multiple cardiac MRI views and train CNNs on related tasks simultaneously for better generalization
	Transfer learning and pretraining	Pretraining on large datasets like ImageNet accelerates learning and improves performance
	Ensemble methods	Combine predictions from multiple models for enhanced robustness and accuracy
	Attention mechanisms	Direct focus on critical heart regions, improving accuracy and interpretability
Case study: Automatic left ventricle segmentation and ejection fraction calculation	Data acquisition	Collect short-axis MRI slices over the cardiac cycle with manual segmentation as ground truth
	Model architecture	Use 2D U-net for frame-by-frame segmentation; 3D U-net for contextual data
	Training strategy	Train on annotated masks with data augmentation and loss functions like dice loss
	Segmentation inference	Predict masks for slices and frames; calculate heart volumes at end-diastole and end-systole
	Ejection fraction calculation	Compute ejection fraction from volume differences, achieving near-expert performance with CNN-based segmentation

Through a combination of these layers, CNNs have demonstrated incredible capabilities in standard image recognition tasks. Transferring these capabilities to the medical domain—particularly in cardiac MRI analysis—requires adapting CNN architectures to the intricacies of medical data, dealing with class imbalance, and leveraging specialized loss functions or training strategies that target clinically relevant metrics.

2.4.2 Applying CNNs to Cardiac MRI

Cardiac MRI presents a rich and challenging dataset. Each scan typically consists of multiple slices covering the heart in different views (short-axis, four-chamber, and two-chamber views) and across multiple time frames throughout the cardiac cycle. Moreover, clinicians are often interested in precise measurements such as left ventricular volume and myocardial thickness, which require accurately segmenting the heart's anatomical structures. Below are some of the key ways CNNs are leveraged in cardiac MRI analysis (Table 2.2):

I. ***Segmentation of Cardiac Structures:*** One of the primary tasks in cardiac MRI is segmenting the ventricles, myocardium, and other structures. Accurate segmentation is essential for measuring ejection fraction, assessing wall motion abnormalities, and quantifying myocardial mass. CNNs, particularly variants like the U-Net architecture, have become standard for medical image segmentation. They employ an encoder-decoder structure that captures both local features (via convolutions) and global context (through upsampling paths that combine coarse and fine features) [75].

II. ***Automated Diagnosis:*** Beyond Segmentation, CNNs can be trained to detect specific cardiac conditions. For instance, CNNs can classify whether a patient's MRI shows signs of hypertrophic cardiomyopathy, ischemic heart disease, or myocarditis [76]. By training on a large labeled dataset, CNN models can learn subtle patterns indicative of a specific pathology [77]. This can help clinicians make faster and more accurate diagnoses, especially when radiologists or cardiologists face heavy workloads.

III. ***Functional Parameter Estimation:*** Cardiac functional parameters such as stroke volume, ejection fraction, and diastolic function are vital to understanding heart performance [78]. CNNs can facilitate the automated computation of these parameters by segmenting cardiac chambers across each frame in the cardiac cycle [75, 79]. The model can track the heart's movement across these frames, enabling volume calculations that reveal how efficiently the heart pumps blood.

IV. ***Feature Extraction for Prognostic Modeling:*** CNNs can also serve as feature extractors. The final layer(s) can provide a compact, high-level feature representation of the images by training or fine-tuning a CNN on a cardiac MRI dataset [80]. These features can then be used in downstream tasks like survival analysis or risk stratification for heart failure. This approach can reduce the reliance on manually engineered features by letting the CNN learn patterns more directly correlated with clinical outcomes [80].

2.4.3 Key Challenges in CNN-Based Cardiac MRI Analysis

Despite the promise of CNNs, applying them to cardiac MRI introduces several challenges [81, 82] (Table 2.2).

I. ***Limited and Imbalanced Datasets:*** Obtaining large, well-labeled cardiac MRI datasets can be difficult. In many medical imaging tasks, labels require expert annotation, which is time-consuming and expensive. Moreover, particular diseases may be rare, creating imbalanced datasets. CNNs trained on such datasets risk overfitting or learning biases toward the majority class. Techniques such as data augmentation, synthetic data generation (using GAN, for instance), and transfer learning from large natural image datasets can help alleviate these challenges.

II. ***Variability in Image Acquisition:*** Cardiac MRI protocols can differ widely across institutions, scanners, and patient conditions. Variations in slice orientation, image resolution, and contrast settings can affect CNN performance. Robust data normalization and domain adaptation techniques may be necessary to ensure that models generalize to new clinical settings [83].

III. ***Temporal Component:*** Cardiac MRI often includes a time series of images that capture cardiac motion. Traditional CNNs process images in a static manner. While 2D CNNs can be extended to 3D CNNs (adding a dimension for slices) or 2.5D approaches (combining adjacent slices for context), fully capturing temporal information may require 4D modeling (three spatial dimensions plus time) [84]. This significantly increases the computational and memory requirements, making model training more challenging.

IV. ***Explainability and Trust:*** In medical applications, explainability is paramount. Clinicians need to understand how a CNN arrived at a particular diagnosis. Current research focuses on saliency maps, class activation maps, and other explainable AI methods to visually explain which parts of the image contributed most to a model's decision. Fostering trust in these models is essential for widespread clinical adoption [85].

V. ***Regulatory and Ethical Considerations:*** Models used for clinical decision-making must adhere to stringent regulatory requirements. They also raise ethical questions about data privacy, informed consent, and potential biases [86]. Any CNN-based system intended for patient care must undergo rigorous validation to ensure reliability and safety [87].

2.4.4 Techniques and Advances for Improved CNN Performance

Over the past decade, researchers have introduced a myriad of techniques and architectural improvements to make CNNs more efficient, robust, and accurate for cardiac MRI tasks:

I. ***U-Net and Variants:*** The U-Net architecture, originally developed for biomedical image segmentation, has become one of the most popular CNN architectures in medical imaging. Its symmetrical encoder-decoder structure and skip connections preserve high-resolution feature information. Variants such as V-Net, Attention U-Net, and UNet++ introduce improvements like 3D convolutions, attention mechanisms, or more sophisticated skip connection strategies to enhance segmentation performance [88–90].

II. ***Multi-View and Multi-Task Learning:*** In cardiac MRI, it is common to have multiple views (short-axis, four-chamber, and two-chamber) that provide complementary information. Multi-view CNNs can learn from all these views simultaneously, improving overall accuracy and robustness [91]. Multi-task learning—where a single CNN is trained to perform multiple related tasks, such as segmentation and classification—can lead to better generalization by sharing learned features across tasks [92].

III. ***Transfer Learning and Pretraining:*** Due to the relative scarcity of large labeled medical image datasets, transfer learning techniques are popular [93, 94]. Models can be pretrained on large natural image datasets (such as ImageNet), and then fine-tuned on cardiac MRI images. Although there is a domain gap between natural images and MRI scans, pretraining often accelerates convergence and improves performance, especially when data are limited [9, 83].

IV. ***Ensemble Methods:*** Combining multiple CNN models via ensembling can boost predictive performance and reduce variance. Different CNN architectures might capture different aspects of the image, and averaging or voting on their predictions often yields more robust results [85, 95]. Ensembling can be computationally expensive, but the accuracy gains may be worthwhile in safety-critical applications like cardiac diagnostics [96].

V. ***Attention Mechanisms:*** Attention modules can direct the CNN's focus to the most relevant regions of the image. In cardiac MRI, certain slices or time frames may be more informative about a condition [97, 98]. By learning attention weights, CNN can prioritize important features and ignore the noise. This improves accuracy and enhances interpretability by highlighting the heart regions the model deems most relevant [98].

2.4.5 Case Study: Automatic Left Ventricle Segmentation and Ejection Fraction Calculation

A representative example of CNN-based analysis in cardiac MRI is automatic left ventricle (LV) segmentation and subsequent ejection fraction calculation. The left ventricle is arguably the most critical cardiac structure for overall pumping function, and its ejection fraction is a key clinical marker (Table 2.2).

I. ***Data Acquisition:*** A dataset of short-axis MRI slices spanning the full cardiac cycle is typically collected. The ground truth consists of manual segmentations of the left ventricle across each time frame.

II. ***Model Architecture:*** A popular choice is a 2D U-Net, processing each slice frame-by-frame. If 3D context is needed, a 3D U-Net can be used, but it requires greater computational resources.

III. ***Training Strategy:*** The network is trained on segmentation masks provided by expert annotators. Loss functions like Dice loss or cross-entropy loss are standard. Data augmentation can increase robustness by adding rotations, shifts, and intensity perturbations.

IV. ***Segmentation Inference:*** The model predicts segmentation masks for each slice and time frame in new images after training. The segmented left ventricle region is then used to calculate the volume at both end-diastole (maximum volume) and end-systole (minimum volume).

V. ***Ejection Fraction Calculation:*** The difference between end-diastolic volume and end-systolic volume divided by end-diastolic volume provides the ejection fraction. CNN-based segmentation has been shown to achieve near-expert performance, significantly reducing analysis time.

This workflow dramatically streamlines clinical routines. Instead of manually delineating the heart in each frame—a laborious process—clinicians can rely on rapid, fully automated methods. Such automation paves the way for real-time or near-real-time cardiac function assessment, thereby improving patient care.

2.5 Image Preprocessing: Enhancing MRI Image Quality for

CMR is deemed the gold standard for cardiac function assessment, given its ability to comprehensively evaluate cardiac morphology, function, and myocardial perfusion [52, 99]. DL—through feature extraction and pattern recognition without manually determining features—in conjunction with proper data preprocessing, enables a highly efficient interpretation of the CMR [52, 100]. While DL algorithms outperform former ML models, they profoundly depend on large sample sizes to prevent overfitting—being well-fitted to the training set while not generalizable to the test set or a new dataset [101]. Medical images—especially CMR—are among the most costly modalities in data acquisition, and preparing a well-annotated large-scale data set is typically not feasible given its high cost and time-consuming annotation [102].

Enhancing the generalizability of the trained model is of utmost importance. Attempts to improve the generalizability of deep-learning MRI segmentation models have suggested that efficient and elegant preprocessing could be more fruitful than only modifying the neural network's architecture. Data preprocessing facilitates the model's training [103].

2.5.1 Resampling and Resizing

MRI images captured using different scanners and protocols can cause the 3D pixels, or voxels, to have unequal spacing in different directions [103, 104]. This inconsistency hinders the DL model from recognizing patterns accurately since the geometry of the voxels is not uniform across the dataset, and the training model does not natively acknowledge voxel spacing [103, 104]. To address this shortcoming, it is suggested that the images and their labeled masks be resampled to maintain a consistent voxel size and align them with the median voxel spacing from the training data [103, 104]. For the segmentation masks, the nearest-neighbor interpolation could be deployed, preserving the integrity of the labels [103, 104]. A smoother approach for the images, e.g., third-order spline interpolation, ensures minimal loss of the important details [103, 104]. Finally, using bicubic interpolation to fine-tune the images further in the areas with higher resolution keeps them as clear and accurate as possible. This process helps ensure the CNNs have uniform and reliable data to learn from, improving their ability to recognize anatomical structures [103].

Different MRI scanners produce variable image shapes. Despite that, the resampling—altering the voxel spacings—could also introduce shape inconsistency to the dataset [103]. Therefore, homogenizing the size of images—e.g., resizing to the median shape of the data set—using padding and cropping is essential to prevent information loss before training [103] (Table 2.3).

2.5.2 Normalization

The image intensity variation of MRI hinders consistent interpretation to the extent to which the repeated MRI of a single patient with the same scanner and same protocol might differ, given the scanner-associated factors [105]. Nyúl

Table 2.3 Image preprocessing for enhancing MRI quality

Process	Key techniques	Purpose	Key insights
Resampling and resizing	- resampling to median voxel size- nearest-neighbor interpolation (masks)- Bicubic interpolation (images)- padding and cropping for size consistency	Ensures uniform voxel geometry and size consistency across data	Improves CNNs' ability to learn from consistent and accurate data [76, 77]
Normalization	- intensity normalization- batch normalization- perturbed normalization	Reduces intensity and parameter variation	Alleviates scanner-related heterogeneity and improves model training stability [78–83]
Data augmentation	**I. Basic augmentation:**- geometric transformations- Mixup **II. Deformable augmentation:**- random displacement fields- spline interpolation- deformable image registration- statistical shape models- contour augmentation **III. Deep Learning-based augmentation:** GANs (e.g., Pix2Pix, CycleGAN, StitchGAN)	Expands training set diversity and size	Enhances generalizability and robustness of models, especially in datasets with high variability [74–110]
Reconstruction	- SANTIS- k-space model of movement artifacts- spline interpolation- CycleGAN- N4ITK bias field correction	Mitigates sampling inconsistencies, noise, and artifacts	Enables high-quality image synthesis and artifact correction [74, 90–113]

et al. introduced an intensity normalization technique to homogenize the intensity interpretation across patients and acquisitions, using intensity landmarks [105, 106]. Thus, the intensity normalization enhanced the trained model's performance by alleviating the heterogeneity of MRI acquisition [106].

The distributions of DL model parameters change as the layers get deeper, and each parameter is under the influence of all its preceding parameters; therefore, hyperparameters are determined carefully, especially the learning rate [107]. Alterations in the distribution of the input layer result in a "covariate shift" [107–109]. Adding a normalization layer between all layers of the DL model—known as Batch Normalization—addresses this shortcoming through internal covariate shift reduction [107]. Normalizing each layer's parameter scale enables deploying higher learning rates without the risk of divergence [107, 109].

Perturbed normalization randomly changes the target mean and standard deviation used in the standard normalization and subsequently changes normalization target parameters for each iteration. The perturbed normalization could outperform the batch normalization [110] (Table 2.3).

2.5.3 Data Augmentation

Data augmentation is one of the most valuable techniques for increasing the sample size and training set diversity when collecting large-scale data sets is not feasible [101, 102].

Data augmentation uses the available training set to generate new observations by applying various modifications to the training set observations—leaving the observation's label unchanged. By expanding the training set's scale and diversity, data augmentation enhances the generalizability of the DL model [102, 111–113]. Currently, three primary augmentation methods are available, i.e., basic, deformable, and DL-based image augmentation [101, 102] (Table 2.3).

2.5.3.1 Basic Augmentation

As suggested by its name, basic augmentations typically encompass sampling, geometric adjustments, and color transformations and are computed fast [101, 102]. Geometric transformation—encompassing translation, flipping, scaling, skewing, shearing, and rotation—is the predominant basic augmentation method employed. The geometric transformation could be used either manually or randomly, and it could be used in conjunction with another [101]. Cropping, occlusion, noise injection, intensity modification, and filtering are among other types of geometric transformations [101]. Using these geometric transformations in conjunction attains higher accuracy compared to employing each alone [110]. Mixup in another transformation generates new observations through a convex combination of training data and their respective labels. This method favors between-training linear behavior and enhances the robustness of the model to overfitting [114]. Mixup outperforms conventional methods in practice as well [115]. Basic augmentations are not intended to generate realistic observations; rather, they aim to enhance the learning of the general [101].

2.5.3.2 Deformable Augmentation

Deformable augmentation provides enhanced variability—improving the generalizability of the model—when the basic methods are incapable of providing sufficient variability [101]. The randomized displacement field is a deformable augmentation technique, displacing each pixel with a random value within the $(-1,1)$ range on the vertical and horizontal axis. The standard deviation of the Gaussian that convolves Δx and Δy determines the smoothness of the deformation. This method increases shape variations to augment the training set [101, 116]. Spline interpolation is another approach to deformable augmentation in which local polynomial interpolation is performed using various interpolation methods, e.g., B-spline interpolation and thin plate spline interpolation [101]. Notably, the utilities of spline interpolation are not constrained to data augmentation. It also enhances image quality, reduces artifacts, and uses dose-reduction imaging techniques [101, 117–119].

Deformable image registration is a registration-based augmentation method that considers one image as the reference (fixed) and tries to increase the similarity of another image (moving) to the reference. One of the methods to augment training data for models designed to detect lesions is adding lesions to the imaging of healthy patients by deformable image registration [120]. The reference image could also be chosen from a template, or two lesioned images could be registered together to generate a new image [101, 121, 122]. Using statistical shape models enables the generation of deformations confined to the variability of ground-truth observation—by designing a statistical model capturing the shape variability within the dataset. Moreover, the statistical shape models result in non-affine and anatomically plausible deformations [123]. As described by Acero et al. [123], taking advantage of the statistical shape model along with other augmentation methods enhances endocardium and myocardium segmentation performance on the CMR compared to not using augmentation; however, this superiority started to diminish as the size of the training increased. The size of the training set is one of the critical determinants of data augmentation's impact on performance [123]. Additionally, the advantages of these augmentations were more pronounced when the model was trained on data sets with high data variability, as in Hypertrophic Cardiomyopathy (HCM) patients [123].

Accurate labeling and annotation are the cornerstone of a sufficient deep-learning segmentation model. However, inter- and intra-observer variability is inevitable in manual annotations [101, 124]. Contour augmentation is another deformable augmentation introduced to remedy this concern [124]. Contour augmentations in combination with data augmentation outperform each alone and not augmentation dataset. The contour augmentation enabled the trained model to adjust for slight offsets of ground truth annotations, thus training a more robust model to inter- and intra-observer variability of the ground truth [124].

2.5.3.3 Deep Learning-Based Augmentation

DL models could also be employed in the preprocessing step of training another DL model; however, they have a relatively high computation cost [101]. One of the most common DL -based augmentations is the GAN, which consists of two adversarial DL multilayer models; one is the generative model designed to synthesize new images, and the other model is the discriminative model aimed at determining whether the generative model generates a specific image or is ground truth. These two models continue to enhance their performance until the discriminative model cannot distinguish generated images from the ground truth—reaching a 50% probability for the discriminative model to determine whether an image is ground truth or generative [101, 125, 126]. The synthesized images are thus plausible in the real world, for they are tested against ground truth [101, 125].

Conditional GAN conditions both generative and discriminative mode and their outputs, increasing the quality and plausibility of the generated images [101, 127]. For instance, including SPatially-Adaptive (DE)normalization layers (SPADE) within the generative model—a condition to be included in the GAN—is shown to preserve the semantic segmentation's anatomy when training a model on CMR; thus, the generated images are more realistic [128–130].

Pix2Pix GAN is another conditional GAN that uses U-Net as the generative model. Requiring a large sample of a paired data set is the primary concern hindering the utilization of Pix2Pix GAN [131]. Other conditional GAN-based augmentation methods overcoming this obstacle are DualGAN, DiscoGAN, and Cycle Consistent GAN (CycleGAN) [131]. CycleGAN is a conditional GAN with its condition being "cycle consistency," meaning the generated image should be reversible to the original one [132]. The CycleGAN is not only employed for augmentation; it has been used for image reconstruction and dose reduction of CT scans [132–135].

The StitchGAN breaks down the complex task of generating an entire image into simpler tasks of sub-image synthesis, and using the StitchLayer generates a whole image by combining these sub-images. The StitchGAN has reduced overfitting and enhanced diversity for multi-parametric MRI synthesis [131]. The Capsule Network-Based GAN (CapGAN) uses a capsule network for the discriminative model of its GAN. The images synthesized by CapGan yielded higher quality and were more realistic than GANs [136]. The Sketching-Rendering Unconditional GAN (SkrGAN), as suggested by its name, is an unconditional GAN. The SkrGAN is composed of two modules, one to sketch the constraints of structures from random noise, completed by the second module, and designed to render color images respecting the structures generated by the first module. The advantage of SkrGAN is that it respects the foreground structures and generates realistic foreground structures [137]. The Texture-Constrained Multichannel Progressive GAN (TMP-GAN) deploys texture discrimination loss, enhancing texture continuity. Therefore, TMP-GAN is well-suited for delicate texture imaging [112].

2.5.4 Reconstruction

The Sampling-Augmented Neural neTwork with Incoherent Structure (SANTIS) is a deep-learning-based method to reconstruct MRI, reduce sampling inconsistency, and omit undersampling artefacts [138]. The k-Space Model of Movement Artefacts is designed to introduce plausible movement artifacts to MRI free of artifacts, enabling the DL model to train on augmented data sets with more variability, thus attaining enhanced generalizability. The k-Space Model of Movement Artefacts could also retrospectively remove movement artifacts from the ground truth [139].

Some image synthesis techniques could also generate a part of the image to reconstruct the original image and omit noise, improve quality, and omit artifacts. As discussed above, the spline interpolation is one of these techniques [101, 117–119]. The CycleGAN is another augmentation technique capable of image reconstruction and CT scan dose reduction [132–135]. The nonparametric nonuniform intensity normalization (N3) was an algorithm previously employed to enhance the MRI quality and reduce its inhomogeneity. Subsequently, a more efficient algorithm named N4ITK was introduced, which was based on N3 with the addition of a robust B-spline approximation in the algorithm. The B-spline enables the algorithm to perform more accurate and smoother bias field correction. Moreover, the N4ITK has a modified optimization approach, which allows for iterative and incremental adjustments to the bias field and consequently enhances the convergence performance compared to N3 [140] (Table 2.3).

This table captures the essence of the techniques, their purpose, and their specific applications, offering a structured summary for efficient understanding.

2.6 Upcoming Strategies and Future Directions

As cardiac imaging continues to evolve, CNNs will likely remain a core technology. Several promising directions are emerging:

Integration with Other Modalities: Often, clinicians have access to multiple imaging modalities, such as echocardiography or CT, in addition to MRI. CNNs that integrate these heterogeneous data sources—sometimes called multimodal learning—have the potential to yield more comprehensive diagnostic insights.

4D Modeling and Motion Analysis: Cardiac MRI data are inherently 4D (3D + time). Many CNN applications flatten the time dimension or treat the data slice-by-slice. More advanced architectures that explicitly capture temporal dynamics—e.g., using RNN or spatiotemporal convolutions—could provide deeper insight into cardiac function.

Real-Time Deployment: With hardware acceleration (e.g., using GPUs or specialized AI chips), CNN inference can be performed quickly. As these devices become more compact and integrated into clinical workflows, real-time analysis of cardiac MRI scans could assist clinicians during or immediately after imaging, speeding up diagnosis and intervention.

Explainable AI: Efforts to enhance the transparency and interpretability of CNNs remain a top priority in medicine. Future research may provide standardized frameworks for explaining CNN decisions, from highlighting key image regions to providing textual justifications. Such capabilities are essential for regulatory approvals and clinician acceptance.

Federated Learning: Privacy concerns and regulations often prevent large-scale data sharing across institutions. Federated learning enables CNNs to train on decentralized data without transferring patient information to a central server. This technique could yield more generalized and robust models while respecting patient privacy regulations.

2.7 Conclusion

CNNs have undoubtedly transformed image recognition across a vast array of domains, and their impact on cardiac MRI analysis is equally significant. By leveraging their ability to learn nuanced, hierarchical features directly from raw images, CNNs can outperform many traditional approaches that depend on engineered features and heuristics. In cardiology, tasks like anatomical segmentation, disease classification, and functional parameter estimation benefit from the precision and efficiency of these DL models.

However, building and deploying CNN-based systems for cardiac MRI is not without its hurdles. Issues such as small datasets, domain variability, and the need for model explainability are critical. Researchers have responded with various innovative strategies, ranging from data augmentation and transfer learning to advanced architectures, such as U-Net and attention-based networks. Future advancements are poised further to enhance reliability, interpretability, and clinical integration, bolstering CNNs' role in cardiac care.

Ultimately, the progress in CNN-driven cardiac MRI analysis exemplifies the broader revolution of AI in healthcare. As more data become available, computational resources continue to grow, and researchers refine model architectures, one can expect CNNs to deliver increasingly detailed and accurate insights into the heart's structure and function. This, in turn, will improve the early detection of disease, facilitate more precise treatment planning, and possibly lead to better patient outcomes. The era of intelligent, data-driven cardiology is well underway, and CNNs stand at the forefront of this transformative wave.

References

1. Alowais SA, et al. Revolutionizing healthcare: the role of artificial intelligence in clinical practice. BMC Med Educ. 2023;23(1):689.
2. Davenport T, Kalakota R. The potential for artificial intelligence in healthcare. Future Healthc J. 2019;6(2):94–8.
3. Lin A, et al. Artificial intelligence: improving the efficiency of cardiovascular imaging. Expert Rev Med Devices. 2020;17(6):565–77.
4. Ledziński Ł, Grześk G. Artificial intelligence technologies in cardiology. J Cardiovasc Dev Dis. 2023;10(5):202.
5. Mathur P, et al. Artificial intelligence, machine learning, and cardiovascular disease. Clin Med Insights Cardiol. 2020;14:1179546820927404.
6. Krittanawong C, et al. Artificial intelligence in precision cardiovascular medicine. J Am Coll Cardiol. 2017;69(21):2657–64.
7. Johnson KW, et al. Artificial intelligence in cardiology. J Am Coll Cardiol. 2018;71(23):2668–79.
8. Young T, et al. Recent trends in deep learning based natural language processing. IEEE Comput Intell Mag. 2018;13(3):55–75.
9. Alzubaidi L, et al. MedNet: pre-trained convolutional neural network model for the medical imaging tasks. arXiv preprint arXiv:2110.06512. 2021;
10. Laranjo L, et al. Conversational agents in healthcare: a systematic review. J Am Med Inform Assoc. 2018;25(9):1248–58.
11. Duchateau N, King AP. AI and Big Data in cardiology.
12. Lin X, Li X, Lin X. A review on applications of computational methods in drug screening and design. Molecules. 2020;25(6):1375.
13. Badura A, et al. Application of artificial neural networks to prediction of new substances with antimicrobial activity against Escherichia coli. J Appl Microbiol. 2021;130(1):40–9.
14. Seetharam K, Min JK. Artificial intelligence and machine learning in cardiovascular imaging. Methodist Debakey Cardiovasc J. 2020;16(4):263.
15. He B, et al. Blinded, randomized trial of sonographer versus AI cardiac function assessment. Nature. 2023;616(7957):520–4.
16. Moghaddasi H, Nourian S. Automatic assessment of mitral regurgitation severity based on extensive textural features on 2D echocardiography videos. Comput Biol Med. 2016;73:47–55.
17. Sengupta PP, et al. Cognitive machine-learning algorithm for cardiac imaging: a pilot study for differentiating constrictive pericarditis from restrictive cardiomyopathy. Circ Cardiovasc Imaging. 2016;9(6):e004330.
18. Opincariu D, et al. From CT to artificial intelligence for complex assessment of plaque-associated risk. Int J Cardiovasc Imaging. 2020;36(12):2403–27.
19. Tatsugami F, et al. Recent advances in artificial intelligence for cardiac CT: enhancing diagnosis and prognosis prediction. Diagn Interv Imaging. 2023;
20. Oksuz I, et al. Automatic CNN-based detection of cardiac MR motion artefacts using k-space data augmentation and curriculum learning. Med Image Anal. 2019;55:136–47.
21. Davies RH, et al. Precision measurement of cardiac structure and function in cardiovascular magnetic resonance using machine learning. J Cardiovasc Magn Reson. 2022;24(1):16.
22. Koulaouzidis G, et al. Artificial intelligence in cardiology—a narrative review of current status. J Clin Med. 2022;11(13):3910.
23. Arsanjani R, et al. Prediction of revascularization after myocardial perfusion SPECT by machine learning in a large population. J Nucl Cardiol. 2015;22(5):877–84.
24. Perez MV, et al. Large-scale assessment of a smartwatch to identify atrial fibrillation. N Engl J Med. 2019;381(20):1909–17.
25. Gupta MD, et al. Artificial intelligence in cardiology: the past, present and future. Indian Heart J. 2022;74(4):265–9.
26. Lim LJ, Tison GH, Delling FN. Artificial intelligence in cardiovascular imaging. Methodist Debakey Cardiovasc J. 2020;16(2):138.
27. Rajoub B. Chapter 3: Supervised and unsupervised learning. In: Zgallai W, editor. Biomedical signal processing and artificial intelligence in healthcare. Academic Press; 2020. p. 51–89.
28. Geetha G, et al. Deep learning with unsupervised and supervised approaches in medical image analysis. In: 2022 2nd international conference on advance computing and innovative technologies in engineering (ICACITE); 2022.
29. Madhushani A. Supervised and unsupervised learning (machine learning). AI and Machine Learning; 2022.
30. Tishan Y. Understanding the difference between supervised and unsupervised Learning techniques; 2023.
31. Elahi R, Nazari M. An updated overview of radiomics-based artificial intelligence (AI) methods in breast cancer screening and diagnosis. arXiv preprint arXiv:2406.14735. 2024;

32. Sathya R, Abraham A. Comparison of supervised and unsupervised learning algorithms for pattern classification. Int J Adv Res Artif Intell. 2013;2(2):34–8.
33. Richards JA, Richards JA. Clustering and unsupervised classification. Remote Sens Digit Image Anal. 2022:369–401.
34. Benčević M, et al. Self-supervised learning as a means to reduce the need for labeled data in medical image analysis. In: 2022 30th European Signal Processing Conference (EUSIPCO); 2022.
35. Bai W, et al. Self-supervised learning for cardiac MR image segmentation by anatomical position prediction. In: Medical image computing and computer assisted intervention—MICCAI 2019, 2019. Cham: Springer.
36. Ackl N, et al. Hippocampal metabolic abnormalities in mild cognitive impairment and Alzheimer's disease. Neurosci Lett. 2005;384(1–2):23–8.
37. Schlemper J, et al. A deep Cascade of convolutional neural networks for dynamic MR image reconstruction. IEEE Trans Med Imaging. 2018;37(2):491–503.
38. Bernard O, et al. Deep Learning techniques for automatic MRI cardiac multi-structures segmentation and diagnosis: is the problem solved? IEEE Trans Med Imaging. 2018;37(11):2514–25.
39. Romaguera L, et al. Myocardial segmentation in cardiac magnetic resonance images using fully convolutional neural networks. Biomed Signal Process Control. 2017;44
40. Winther HB, et al. ν-net: deep Learning for generalized biventricular mass and function parameters using multicenter cardiac MRI data. JACC Cardiovasc Imaging. 2018;11(7):1036–8.
41. Tan LK, et al. Convolutional neural network regression for short-axis left ventricle segmentation in cardiac cine MR sequences. Med Image Anal. 2017;39:78–86.
42. Otazo R, et al. Combination of compressed sensing and parallel imaging for highly accelerated first-pass cardiac perfusion MRI. Magn Reson Med. 2010;64(3):767–76.
43. Chen X, et al. Accelerated two-dimensional cine DENSE cardiovascular magnetic resonance using compressed sensing and parallel imaging. J Cardiovasc Magn Reson. 2016;18(1):38.
44. Oksuz I, et al. Unsupervised myocardial Segmentation for cardiac BOLD. IEEE Trans Med Imaging. 2017;36(11):2228–38.
45. Hayes C, et al. Fully automatic planning of the long-axis views of the heart. J Cardiovasc Magn Reson. 2013;15(1):O54.
46. Farrag NA, White JA, Ukwatta E. Semi-automated myocardial segmentation in native T1-mapping CMR using deformable non-rigid registration of CINE images. In: Medical imaging 2019: biomedical applications in molecular, structural, and functional imaging, vol. 10953. SPIE; 2019.
47. Karami P, Elahi R. Radiomics-based artificial intelligence (AI) models in colorectal cancer (CRC) diagnosis, metastasis detection, prognosis, and treatment response. arXiv preprint arXiv:2406.12467. 2024;
48. Baeßler B, et al. Texture analysis and machine learning of non-contrast T1-weighted MR images in patients with hypertrophic cardiomyopathy-preliminary results. Eur J Radiol. 2018;102:61–7.
49. Schofield R, et al. Texture analysis of cardiovascular magnetic resonance cine images differentiates aetiologies of left ventricular hypertrophy. Clin Radiol. 2019;74(2):140–9.
50. Larroza A, et al. Texture analysis of cardiac cine magnetic resonance imaging to detect nonviable segments in patients with chronic myocardial infarction. Med Phys. 2018;45(4):1471–80.
51. Peng F, et al. Magnetic resonance texture analysis in myocardial infarction. Front Cardiovasc Med. 2021;8:724271.
52. Wang Y-R, et al. Screening and diagnosis of cardiovascular disease using artificial intelligence-enabled cardiac magnetic resonance imaging. Nat Med. 2024;30(5):1471–80.
53. Jang J, et al. Sensitivity of myocardial Radiomic features to imaging parameters in cardiac MR imaging. J Magn Reson Imaging. 2021;54(3):787–94.
54. Baessler B, et al. Cardiac MRI texture analysis of T1 and T2 maps in patients with Infarctlike acute myocarditis. Radiology. 2018;289(2):357–65.
55. Kotu LP, et al. Cardiac magnetic resonance image-based classification of the risk of arrhythmias in post-myocardial infarction patients. Artif Intell Med. 2015;64(3):205–15.
56. Zhang N, et al. Deep learning for diagnosis of chronic myocardial infarction on nonenhanced cardiac cine MRI. Radiology. 2019;291(3):606–17.
57. Neisius U, et al. Radiomic analysis of myocardial native T(1) imaging discriminates between hypertensive heart disease and hypertrophic cardiomyopathy. JACC Cardiovasc Imaging. 2019;12(10):1946–54.
58. Fahmy AS, et al. Automated analysis of cardiovascular magnetic resonance myocardial native T1 mapping images using fully convolutional neural networks. J Cardiovasc Magn Reson. 2019;21(1):7.
59. Swift AJ, et al. A machine learning cardiac magnetic resonance approach to extract disease features and automate pulmonary arterial hypertension diagnosis. Eur Heart J Cardiovasc Imaging. 2021;22(2):236–45.
60. Ambale-Venkatesh B, et al. Cardiovascular event prediction by machine learning: the multi-ethnic study of atherosclerosis. Circ Res. 2017;121(9):1092–101.
61. King B, et al. Unsupervised clustering of COVID-19 chest X-Ray images with a self-organizing feature map. In: 2020 IEEE 63rd international midwest symposium on circuits and systems (MWSCAS). IEEE; 2020. p. 395–8.

62. Casaclang-Verzosa G, et al. Network tomography for understanding phenotypic presentations in aortic stenosis. JACC Cardiovasc Imaging. 2019;12(2):236–48.
63. Mukhopadhyay A, et al. Unsupervised myocardial segmentation for cardiac MRI. In: Medical image computing and computer-assisted intervention—MICCAI. Cham: Springer; 2015.
64. Granizo S, et al. A comparative analysis of vision transformers and convolutional neural networks in cardiac image segmentation. In: 2024 12th international symposium on digital forensics and security (ISDFS). IEEE; 2024.
65. Duong SQ, et al. Ensemble modeling of multimodal electrocardiogram and echocardiogram data improves quantitative assessment of right ventricular function. JACC Adv. 2024;3(9):101186.
66. Siegel EL, Morris M. Artificial intelligence in nuclear medicine: counterpoint—more hype than reality today. Am J Roentgenol. 2024;223(4):e2431299.
67. Pham TV, et al. CapNet: an automatic attention-based with mixer model for cardiovascular magnetic resonance image Segmentation. J Imaging Inform Med. 2024:1–30.
68. Li Z, et al. A survey of convolutional neural networks: analysis, applications, and prospects. IEEE Trans. Neural Netw. Learn. Syst. 2021;33(12):6999–7019.
69. Yamashita R, et al. Convolutional neural networks: an overview and application in radiology. Insights Imaging. 2018;9:611–29.
70. Gu J, et al. Recent advances in convolutional neural networks. Pattern Recogn. 2018;77:354–77.
71. Sun M, et al. Learning pooling for convolutional neural network. Neurocomputing. 2017;224:96–104.
72. Basha SS, et al. Impact of fully connected layers on performance of convolutional neural networks for image classification. Neurocomputing. 2020;378:112–9.
73. Qian S, et al. Adaptive activation functions in convolutional neural networks. Neurocomputing. 2018;272:204–12.
74. Santos CFGD, Papa JP. Avoiding overfitting: a survey on regularization methods for convolutional neural networks. ACM Comput Surveys (CSUR). 2022;54(10s):1–25.
75. Zotti C, et al. Convolutional neural network with shape prior applied to cardiac MRI segmentation. IEEE J Biomed Health Inform. 2018;23(3):1119–28.
76. Jafari M, et al. Automated diagnosis of cardiovascular diseases from cardiac magnetic resonance imaging using deep learning models: a review. Comput Biol Med. 2023;160:106998.
77. Agibetov A, et al. Convolutional neural networks for fully automated diagnosis of cardiac amyloidosis by cardiac magnetic resonance imaging. J Pers Med. 2021;11(12):1268.
78. Li T, et al. Direct estimation of left ventricular ejection fraction via a cardiac cycle feature learning architecture. Comput Biol Med. 2020;118:103659.
79. Xue H, et al. Landmark detection in cardiac MRI by using a convolutional neural network. Radiology. 2021;3(5):e200197.
80. Gao Y, et al. Deep learning-based prognostic model using non-enhanced cardiac cine MRI for outcome prediction in patients with heart failure. Eur Radiol. 2023;33(11):8203–13.
81. Bernard O, et al. Deep learning techniques for automatic MRI cardiac multi-structures segmentation and diagnosis: is the problem solved? IEEE Trans Med Imaging. 2018;37(11):2514–25.
82. Rajiah PS, François CJ, Leiner T. Cardiac MRI: state of the art. Radiology. 2023;307(3):e223008.
83. Margeta J, et al. Fine-tuned convolutional neural nets for cardiac MRI acquisition plane recognition. Comput Methods Biomech Biomed Eng Imaging Vis. 2017;5(5):339–49.
84. Patravali J, Jain S, Chilamkurthy S. 2D-3D fully convolutional neural networks for cardiac MR segmentation. In: Statistical atlases and computational models of the heart. ACDC and MMWHS challenges: 8th international workshop, STACOM 2017, held in conjunction with MICCAI 2017, Quebec City, Canada, September 10-14, 2017, revised selected papers 8. Springer; 2018.
85. Ng M, et al. Estimating uncertainty in neural networks for cardiac MRI segmentation: a benchmark study. IEEE Trans Biomed Eng. 2022;70(6):1955–66.
86. Marey A, et al. Applications and implementation of generative artificial intelligence in cardiovascular imaging with a focus on ethical and legal considerations: what cardiovascular imagers need to know! BJR. 2024;1(1):ubae008.
87. Sengupta PP, et al. Challenges for augmenting intelligence in cardiac imaging. Lancet Digit Health. 2024;6(10):e739–48.
88. Wong KK, et al. GCW-UNet segmentation of cardiac magnetic resonance images for evaluation of left atrial enlargement. Comput Methods Prog Biomed. 2022;221:106915.
89. Li W, Wang L, Qin S. CMS-UNet: cardiac multitask segmentation in MRI with a u-shaped network. In: Myocardial pathology segmentation combining multi-sequence cardiac magnetic resonance images: first challenge, MyoPS 2020, held in conjunction with MICCAI 2020, Lima, Peru, October 4, 2020, proceedings 1. Springer; 2020.
90. Kumar R, et al. CBAR-UNet: a novel methodology for segmentation of cardiac magnetic resonance images using block attention-based deep residual neural network. Multimed Tools Appl. 2024:1–17.
91. Mortazi A, et al. CardiacNET: segmentation of left atrium and proximal pulmonary veins from MRI using multi-view CNN. In: Medical image computing and computer-assisted intervention– MICCAI 2017: 20th international conference, Quebec City, QC, Canada, September 11–13, 2017, proceedings, part II 20. Springer; 2017.

92. Duan J, et al. Automatic 3D bi-ventricular segmentation of cardiac images by a shape-refined multi-task deep learning approach. IEEE Trans Med Imaging. 2019;38(9):2151–64.
93. Ho N, Kim Y-C. Evaluation of transfer learning in deep convolutional neural network models for cardiac short axis slice classification. Sci Rep. 2021;11(1):1839.
94. Shin H-C, et al. Deep convolutional neural networks for computer-aided detection: CNN architectures, dataset characteristics and transfer learning. IEEE Trans Med Imaging. 2016;35(5):1285–98.
95. Hann E, et al. Deep neural network ensemble for on-the-fly quality control-driven segmentation of cardiac MRI T1 mapping. Med Image Anal. 2021;71:102029.
96. Aghapanah H, et al. MECardNet: a novel multi-scale convolutional ensemble model with adaptive deep supervision for precise cardiac MRI segmentation. Biomed Signal Process Control. 2025;100:106919.
97. Li Y-Z, et al. RSU-net: U-net based on residual and self-attention mechanism in the segmentation of cardiac magnetic resonance images. Comput Methods Prog Biomed. 2023;231:107437.
98. Zhu D, He H, Wang D. Feedback attention network for cardiac magnetic resonance imaging super-resolution. Comput Methods Prog Biomed. 2023;231:107313.
99. Salerno M, et al. Recent advances in cardiovascular magnetic resonance: techniques and applications. Circulation Cardiovasc Imaging. 2017;10(6):e003951.
100. LeCun Y, Bengio Y, Hinton G. Deep learning. Nature. 2015;521(7553):436–44.
101. Chlap P, et al. A review of medical image data augmentation techniques for deep learning applications. J Med Imaging Radiat Oncol. 2021;65(5):545–63.
102. Chen J, et al. Synchronous medical image augmentation framework for deep learning-based image segmentation. Comput Med Imaging Graph. 2023;104:102161.
103. Khader F, et al. Adaptive preprocessing for generalization in cardiac MR image segmentation. In: Statistical atlases and computational models of the heart. M&Ms and EMIDEC challenges. Cham: Springer; 2021.
104. Isensee F, et al. nnu-net: Self-adapting framework for u-net-based medical image segmentation. arXiv preprint arXiv:1809.10486. 2018;
105. Nyúl LG, Udupa JK, Zhang X. New variants of a method of MRI scale standardization. IEEE Trans Med Imaging. 2000;19(2):143–50.
106. Pereira S, et al. Brain tumor segmentation using convolutional neural networks in MRI images. IEEE Trans Med Imaging. 2016;35(5):1240–51.
107. Ioffe S. Batch normalization: accelerating deep network training by reducing internal covariate shift. arXiv preprint arXiv:1502.03167; 2015.
108. Shimodaira H. Improving predictive inference under covariate shift by weighting the log-likelihood function. J Stat Plann Inference. 2000;90(2):227–44.
109. Curiale AH, et al. Automatic myocardial segmentation by using a deep learning network in cardiac MRI. In: 2017 XLIII Latin American computer conference (CLEI). IEEE; 2017.
110. Kompanek M, Tamajka M, Benesova W. Volumetrie data augmentation as an effective tool in MRI classification using 3D convolutional neural network. In: 2019 international conference on systems, signals and image processing (IWSSIP); 2019.
111. Yang F, et al. Dual attention-guided and learnable spatial transformation data augmentation multi-modal unsupervised medical image segmentation. Biomed Signal Process Control. 2022;78:103849.
112. Guan Q, et al. Medical image augmentation for lesion detection using a texture-constrained multichannel progressive GAN. Comput Biol Med. 2022;145:105444.
113. Chaitanya K, et al. Semi-supervised task-driven data augmentation for medical image segmentation. Med Image Anal. 2021;68:101934.
114. Zhang H. mixup: beyond empirical risk minimization. arXiv preprint arXiv:1710.09412; 2017.
115. Zhao W, et al. Toward automatic prediction of EGFR mutation status in pulmonary adenocarcinoma with 3D deep learning. Cancer Med. 2019;8(7):3532–43.
116. Simard PY, Steinkraus D, Platt JC. Best practices for convolutional neural networks applied to visual document analysis. In: ICDAR. Edinburgh; 2003.
117. Lee H, et al. Low-dose CBCT reconstruction via joint non-local total variation denoising and cubic B-spline interpolation. Sci Rep. 2021;11(1):3681.
118. Verschuur AS, et al. Improved neonatal brain MRI segmentation by interpolation of motion corrupted slices. J Neuroimaging. 2022;32(3):480–92.
119. Scholkmann F, et al. How to detect and reduce movement artifacts in near-infrared imaging using moving standard deviation and spline interpolation. Physiol Meas. 2010;31(5):649–62.
120. Krivov E, Pisov M, Belyaev M. MRI augmentation via elastic registration for brain lesions segmentation. In: Brainlesion: glioma, multiple sclerosis, stroke and traumatic brain injuries. Cham: Springer; 2018.
121. Tustison NJ, et al. Convolutional neural networks with template-based data augmentation for functional lung image quantification. Acad Radiol. 2019;26(3):412–23.
122. Lin D, et al. 2022 IEEE International Conference on Image Processing (ICIP); 2020.
123. Corral Acero J, et al. SMOD—data augmentation based on statistical models of deformation to enhance segmentation. In: 2D cine cardiac MRI. In functional imaging and modeling of the heart. Cham: Springer; 2019.

124. Javaid U, Dasnoy D, Lee JA. Semantic segmentation of computed tomography for radiotherapy with deep learning: compensating insufficient annotation quality using contour augmentation. In: Medical imaging 2019: image processing. SPIE; 2019.
125. Goodfellow I, et al. Generative adversarial nets. Adv Neural Inf Proces Syst. 2014;27
126. Luc P, et al. Semantic segmentation using adversarial networks. arXiv preprint arXiv:1611.08408; 2016.
127. Mirza M, Osindero S. Conditional generative adversarial nets. arXiv preprint arXiv:1411.1784; 2014.
128. Lustermans D, et al. Optimized automated cardiac MR scar quantification with GAN-based data augmentation. Comput Methods Prog Biomed. 2022;226:107116.
129. Abbasi-Sureshjani S, et al. 4D semantic cardiac magnetic resonance image synthesis on XCAT anatomical model. In: Tal A, et al., editors. Proceedings of the third conference on medical imaging with deep learning. PMLR: Proceedings of Machine Learning Research; 2020. p. 6–18.
130. Amirrajab S, et al. XCAT-GAN for synthesizing 3D consistent labeled cardiac MR images on anatomically variable XCAT phantoms. In: Medical image computing and computer assisted intervention—MICCAI. Cham: Springer; 2020.
131. Wang Z, et al. Semi-supervised mp-MRI data synthesis with StitchLayer and auxiliary distance maximization. Med Image Anal. 2020;59:101565.
132. Zhu J-Y, et al. Unpaired image-to-image translation using cycle-consistent adversarial networks. In: Proceedings of the IEEE international conference on computer vision; 2017.
133. Li Y, et al. POCS-augmented CycleGAN for MR image reconstruction. Appl Sci (Basel). 2022;12(1)
134. Cui H, et al. Toward accurate cardiac MRI segmentation with Variational autoencoder-based unsupervised domain adaptation. IEEE Trans Med Imaging. 2024;43(8):2924–36.
135. Gu J, et al. CycleGAN denoising of extreme low-dose cardiac CT using wavelet-assisted noise disentanglement. Med Image Anal. 2021;74:102209.
136. Yu H, Zhang X. Synthesis of prostate MR images for classification using capsule network-based GAN model. Sensors. 2020;20(20):5736.
137. Zhang T, et al. SkrGAN: sketching-rendering unconditional generative adversarial networks for medical image synthesis. In: Medical image computing and computer assisted intervention—MICCAI. Cham: Springer; 2019.
138. Liu F, et al. SANTIS: sampling-augmented neural neTwork with incoherent structure for MR image reconstruction. Magn Reson Med. 2019;82(5):1890–904.
139. Shaw R, et al. A k-space model of movement artefacts: application to segmentation augmentation and artefact removal. IEEE Trans Med Imaging. 2020;39(9):2881–92.
140. Tustison NJ, et al. N4ITK: improved N3 bias correction. IEEE Trans Med Imaging. 2010;29(6):1310–20.

AI-Powered MRI for Precision Diagnosis of Cardiomyopathy: Insights into Hypertrophic, Dilated, Arrhythmogenic, and Restrictive Cardiomyopathies

3

Amir Ghaffari Jolfayi, Mohammadhossein Mozafarybazargany, Hamed Ghoshouni, Elham Shabani, Maedeh Dastmardi, Alireza Salmanipour, and Golnaz Houshmand

Abstract

Cardiovascular diseases, particularly cardiomyopathies, remain leading contributors to global morbidity and mortality, necessitating innovative diagnostic and therapeutic solutions. This chapter explores the transformative potential of Artificial Intelligence (AI) in cardiac magnetic resonance imaging (CMR) for precision diagnosis and management of hypertrophic, dilated, restrictive, and arrhythmogenic cardiomyopathies. CMR is the gold standard for evaluating myocardial structure and function but is often constrained by cost, expertise requirements, and accessibility. AI-driven advancements, including deep learning algorithms, promise to overcome these limitations by automating image analysis, enhancing diagnostic accuracy, and enabling cost-effective non-contrast imaging protocols.

Hypertrophic cardiomyopathy (HCM) benefits from AI-enhanced CMR modalities, such as T1/T2 mapping and cine imaging, for detecting fibrosis and hypertrophy, crucial for sudden cardiac death risk stratification. Similarly, in dilated cardiomyopathy (DCM), AI enables automated segmentation of ventricular structures, precise fibrosis quantification via late gadolinium enhancement (LGE), and improved risk models incorporating clinical and genetic data. For restrictive cardiomyopathy (RCM), AI leverages advanced mapping techniques to differentiate infiltrative and fibrotic pathologies, overcoming diagnostic ambiguities. Arrhythmogenic cardiomyopathy (ACM), characterized by fibrofatty myocardial replacement, sees significant advancements with AI-optimized ECG interpretation and automated CMR segmentation, addressing challenges in phenotypic variability and risk prediction.

Emerging technologies integrated with AI further enhance patient accessibility, reduce

Authors Amir Ghaffari Jolfayi, Mohammadhossein Mozafarybazargany have contributed equality and shared the first co-authorship.

A. Ghaffari Jolfayi · M. Mozafarybazargany
H. Ghoshouni · M. Dastmardi · A. Salmanipour
G. Houshmand (✉)
Cardiovascular Imaging Research Center, Rajaie Cardiovascular Institute, Tehran, Iran

E. Shabani
Clinical Research Development Unit, Mashhad University of Medical Sciences, Mashhad, Iran

A. Ghaffari Jolfayi (ed.), *Navigating Cardiology's Future*,
https://doi.org/10.1007/978-981-95-0313-1_3

costs, and improve scan efficiency. AI's role in standardizing interpretations and supporting personalized medicine underscores its transformative potential. By integrating AI with advanced imaging protocols, this chapter highlights a pathway to scalable, accurate, and patient-centric solutions for managing cardiomyopathies, paving the way for precision cardiology.

Keywords

Cardiac magnetic resonance imaging · Hypertrophic cardiomyopathy · Dilated cardiomyopathy · Arrhythmogenic cardiomyopathy · Restrictive cardiomyopathy · Deep learning · Machine learning · Artificial intelligence

3.1 Hypertrophic Cardiomyopathy (HCM): AI in Detecting Structural Abnormalities and Outcome Prediction

Cardiovascular diseases (CVDs) are a leading cause of premature mortality, with their incidence increasing due to population growth and aging [1, 2]. This trend contributes significantly to escalating healthcare costs and economic burdens. Addressing this challenge necessitates cost-effective and scalable interventions, with Artificial Intelligence (AI) emerging as a crucial tool [3]. Hypertrophic cardiomyopathy (HCM), a prevalent inherited cardiomyopathy, stands out as a major cause of sudden cardiac death (SCD) among young adults. However, effective, scalable solutions for screening this condition remain scarce [4]. HCM is a genetic disorder of the myocardium caused by mutations in genes encoding sarcomeric proteins. It is characterized by pronounced myocardial hypertrophy, myofibrillar disarray, and increased myocardial collagen [5, 6]. The condition affects approximately 1 in 200 individuals worldwide. Early diagnosis of HCM is critical as it enables regular healthcare monitoring, stringent cardiovascular risk management, and the timely initiation of effective risk-reducing therapies [7, 8].

The complex nature of managing HCM can delay decision-making processes. By integrating human expertise with technological advancements, AI offers a solution by streamlining repetitive and time-consuming tasks. This enables physicians to concentrate on patient interaction, judgment, and emotional intelligence, enhancing overall care efficiency [9]. AI can be defined as using computational systems to simulate cognitive functions akin to human intelligence, such as critical thinking and adaptive behavior [10].

Cardiac magnetic resonance (CMR) is the noninvasive reference standard for assessing ventricular volumes. However, it is only available in a few regions [11, 12]. Due to the high cost of technology and the extensive clinical expertise required for its deployment and interpretation, CMR is not a practical option for widespread screening [13, 14]. Nonetheless, it remains a reliable method for diagnosing HCM and is critical for risk stratification regarding SCD [15, 16].

The diagnosis of HCM typically relies on cardiac imaging techniques, including CMR. This technique offers a comprehensive approach to evaluating cardiovascular morphology, ventricular function, myocardial perfusion, tissue characterization, flow quantification, and coronary artery disease [8, 13]. CMR plays an essential role in the diagnosis, risk assessment, and treatment planning for HCM [5]. Our understanding of the clinical utility of cardiac MRI and its imaging phenotypes in cardiomyopathies continues to evolve.

Recently, T1 and T2 mapping sequences have been introduced alongside traditional CMR sequences. These advanced techniques enable a more quantitative evaluation of myocardial changes, such as fibrosis (T1 maps) and edema (T1 and T2 maps). Thus, T1 and T2 mapping have demonstrated significant potential for both diagnostic and prognostic applications in patients with HCM [17].

Native (pre-contrast) CMR modalities provide alternative tissue characterization methods without using gadolinium-based contrast agents

(GBCA). Cine imaging captures a sequence of images across different cardiac phases to evaluate cardiac structure and motion. Native T1 mapping measures tissues' T1 (proton spin-lattice) relaxation time on a pixel-by-pixel basis [18]. This technique is sensitive to various cardiac conditions, including early myocardial alterations seen in HCM [19–21]. Abnormal T1 signals often correlate with areas of late gadolinium enhancement (LGE) and histopathological findings related to focal and diffuse fibrosis [22–24]. Despite its potential, the clinical utility of native T1 mapping has been limited by issues such as a lack of standardized interpretation, variability in postprocessing, and diagnostic specificity. It has been proposed that native T1 maps could be adapted into visually diagnostic images akin to LGE images [18, 25].

Recently, the advancement of AI in non-contrast CMR examination has shown promising results, which can help avoid contrast nephropathy [26–28]. Specifically, machine learning (ML) techniques may eliminate the need for contrast media, thus broadening CMR's clinical applications.

In clinical practice, the rapid increase in CMR examinations calls for optimizing workflows with faster and more cost-effective protocols. Non-contrast CMR examinations, which benefit patients who cannot receive contrast media due to renal disease or other contraindications, offer a shorter image requisition duration and greater patient comfort. This approach not only enhances the accessibility of CMR but also reduces costs and improves patient experience [27, 29]. A study showed that Gadolinium-free approaches (e.g., T1 mapping and cine sequences) are emerging, leveraging AI to avoid contrast-related risks in specific patient populations [27, 30].

The HCM often progresses asymptomatically, but it can occasionally present with ventricular arrhythmias that increase the risk of sudden cardiac death. LGE in cardiac magnetic resonance imaging (CMRI) has been validated to indicate myocardial alterations in HCM patients. The European Society of Cardiology guidelines have noted that LGE correlates with increased cardiovascular morbidity and mortality and serves as a risk factor for non-sustained ventricular tachyarrhythmias in HCM patients. Although these guidelines do not yet recommend using LGE as a definitive risk stratification tool for sudden cardiac death, there is an observed trend indicating a heightened risk. A recent study by Mentias et al. demonstrated the feasibility of using LGE as a surrogate marker for potential sudden cardiac death [5, 31, 32].

LGE-CMR imaging is well-established for identifying focal myocardial lesions and fibrosis across various cardiovascular diseases [33–37]. The extent of LGE is independently linked to adverse outcomes, including in HCM [38–43]. However, LGE requires intravenous administration of GBCA, which poses risks for patients with severe kidney failure or known GBCA allergies [44]. Eliminating the need for GBCA could significantly reduce scan times, lower associated costs, minimize patient preparation, and potentially reduce the need for continuous physician supervision.

As with other imaging modalities, a significant limitation of CMR is the reliance on expert clinician interpretation. The application of AI in cardiac imaging has the potential to enhance the consistency and accuracy of image interpretation. Beyond improving interpretation, AI can streamline the image acquisition process by reducing the time needed to obtain high-quality MRI images and mitigating motion or other artifacts. Ruijsink et al. demonstrated that AI ensures the reliability of CMR outputs by performing pre- and post-analysis quality control, detecting motion artifacts, and ensuring complete LV coverage [45]. Additionally, AI can accelerate the segmentation and reconstruction of MRI data. Recent reviews have detailed the advancements in this evolving field [46]. Some studies have shown that AI, especially deep learning algorithms like U-Net and convolutional neural networks (CNNs), are widely used for automatic LV segmentation. This is critical for measuring key parameters like myocardial thickness, which is a hallmark of HCM [47].

CMR is a critical tool for evaluating cardiomyopathies because it comprehensively assesses ventricular structure and myocardial physiology across various scan planes. The combination of rest and stress myocardial perfusion, regional function analysis, LGE, and T2-weighted imaging helps differentiate the causes of cardiomyopathies and guides management strategies. Recently developed techniques, such as T1 mapping and extracellular volume (ECV) fraction measurement, have provided new diagnostic insights and validated noninvasive estimates of fibrosis or infiltration severity in different cardiomyopathies [48]. Incorporating stress CMR into diagnostic protocols complements LGE imaging by helping exclude ischemia as a contributing factor. Numerous multinational registries now integrate CMR to enhance understanding of genotype-risk interactions in genetic cardiomyopathies [49]. The presence, pattern, and extent of LGE continue to show a strong prognostic association with serious ventricular arrhythmias and sudden cardiac death, although the specific guidelines for implantable cardioverter-defibrillator (ICD) therapy remain under investigation [46, 50].

In a study, an AI model is trained to analyze LV function from cine MRI images, which depict the heart's motion over time. This analysis includes measuring parameters such as LV ejection fraction (LVEF), end-systolic volume (ESV), end-diastolic volume (EDV), and LV mass. These parameters vary significantly between normal, HCM, and DCM patients and help distinguish them [51, 52].

Compared to echocardiography, CMR offers a more comprehensive three-dimensional view of LV hypertrophy and tissue characteristics in patients with HCM. CMR provides greater precision in monitoring disease progression than echocardiography [53]. It is notably more sensitive in diagnosing HCM, capturing details such as hypertrophy of the basal anterior wall or apical aneurysm, which echocardiography may overlook. The LV mass index can vary significantly with the maximum LV wall thickness due to the diverse manifestations of the HCM phenotype. A markedly elevated LV mass index (greater than 91 g/m^2 for men and 69 g/m^2 for women) and a maximal wall thickness exceeding 30 mm are both sensitive and specific indicators of sudden cardiac death risk. In a large series, the extent of LGE has been associated with heterogeneous fibrosis and linked to ventricular arrhythmias, progressive LV dilation, and adverse cardiac events, regardless of the presence of outflow obstruction or previous septal myectomy [32]. CMR's multifaceted approach enables a personalized characterization of abnormal myocardial pathophysiology, including coronary microvascular dysfunction, fibrosis, and hypertrophy. Additionally, cine CMR, LGE, and regional strain imaging can quantify left atrial remodeling and estimate the risk of atrial fibrillation in HCM patients [54, 55].

Recent advancements from specialized centers have demonstrated that myocardial disarray can be visualized using diffusion tensor CMR. The directionality of this disarray, known as fractional anisotropy, has shown a strong association with ventricular arrhythmias independent of fibrosis [56]. The National Heart, Lung, and Blood Institute (NHLBI)-funded HCMR registry has recently completed enrollment of 2755 HCM patients, incorporating CMR, genetic data, biomarker data, and clinical outcomes [57]. Additionally, the large international Sarcomeric Human Cardiomyopathy Registry (SHaRe) includes CMR data to describe the long-term national history of HCM patients with LV dysfunction [58].

Future CMR technology advancements are expected to enhance study throughput, protocol consistency, and patient tolerability. One significant technological breakthrough is compressed sensing, a signal-processing technique introduced in 2004. Compressed sensing demonstrated that digital images could be reconstructed with fewer data samples than traditionally required by Nyquist's Law due to the compressible nature of image information. This technique has shown substantial promise in improving the efficiency of CMR cine, perfusion, 4D flow, and coronary magnetic resonance angiography (MRA) [59]. It facilitates high-quality, real-time imaging of cardiac function without the need for cardiac gating, breath holding, or acquiring whole-heart cine at high resolution in a single breath-hold.

Although MRI technology is generally trending towards higher field strengths to benefit from improved signal-to-noise ratios, low-field CMR (with field strengths less than 1.0T) is under active investigation and has shown promising results in increasing the clinical applicability of CMR. Compared to the conventional 1.5 or 3T MRI systems, low-field CMR offers potential advantages for cardiac patients, including lower scanner and construction costs, more straightforward operation, and reduced heat deposition, making it safer for patients with metallic devices and for claustrophobic patients [60]. The loss in signal-to-noise ratio associated with lower field strengths can be offset by using steady-state free precession (SSFP) methods or optimizing pulse sequence parameters, such as increasing the flip angle, without significantly increasing the risk of tissue heating [61].

In conclusion, HCM, a genetic myocardial disorder and a significant cause of sudden cardiac death, poses diagnostic and management challenges due to its asymptomatic progression and complex phenotype. CMR remains a cornerstone for assessing myocardial structure and function, offering advanced imaging techniques like T1/T2 mapping for fibrosis and edema evaluation. However, the cost and expertise required for traditional contrast-based CMR limit widespread application. AI advancements in non-contrast CMR, leveraging machine learning for automated image interpretation and workflow optimization, promise greater accessibility, cost reduction, and precision. These innovations enhance risk stratification and diagnostic accuracy, particularly in monitoring fibrosis, left ventricular hypertrophy, and arrhythmogenic risk. Emerging technologies, including low-field CMR and compressed sensing, further improve patient tolerability and scanning efficiency, paving the way for personalized HCM care. Integrating AI-driven tools with advancements in CMR can transform HCM management, providing scalable, cost-effective solutions for early diagnosis, risk assessment, and therapy planning.

3.2 Dilated Cardiomyopathy (DCM): Improving Diagnostic Accuracy and Outcome Prediction with AI-Driven MRI

Dilated Cardiomyopathy (DCM) is a form of cardiomyopathy characterized by the dilation and impaired contraction of the heart's ventricles, often leading to systolic dysfunction without significant coronary artery disease, valvular abnormalities, or poorly controlled hypertension [62]. This condition is a significant cause of heart failure and is associated with a high risk of arrhythmias and sudden cardiac death [63]. Traditionally, diagnostic and therapeutic decisions in DCM have been based on clinical findings, echocardiography, and CMR imaging. CMR is often considered the gold standard for evaluating LV volumes, EF, and myocardial tissue characteristics due to its superior spatial resolution and contrast differentiation [64]. However, conventional CMR analysis is limited by manual interpretation, which can be slow, labor-intensive, and prone to inter-observer variability [50].

The advent of AI, particularly ML and DL, is revolutionizing the use of CMR in DCM by automating image analysis, enhancing tissue characterization, and improving risk stratification [65]. AI-driven approaches also allow for integrating diverse data types—imaging, clinical, and genetic—creating opportunities for more personalized medicine [66]. This expanded exploration will delve into the specific mechanisms of AI that enhance CMR for DCM, providing a comprehensive understanding of how AI is reshaping diagnostic and prognostic paradigms in this field.

3.2.1 AI for Automated and Enhanced Image Analysis

CMR imaging provides detailed assessments of the heart's structure and function, making it a valuable tool for diagnosing and managing DCM. Essential parameters such as LV volumes,

EF, and myocardial mass are derived from CMR images [67]. Traditionally, these parameters are calculated through manual or semi-automated segmentation of the heart's chambers, which requires tracing the contours of the endocardial and epicardial borders at specific points in the cardiac cycle (end-diastole and end-systole). This manual segmentation is time-consuming and subject to operator variability, potentially leading to inconsistencies in measurements across different institutions or even between different operators within the same institution [68] [Fig. 3.1].

AI, particularly DL algorithms, is revolutionizing this process by offering fully automated and highly accurate segmentation of the heart's chambers. These DL models are trained on large datasets of annotated CMR images, learning to identify the key anatomical structures of the heart. After training, these models can automatically and accurately delineate the LV, RV, and myocardium across multiple slices and phases of the cardiac cycle [69]. The automation extends to dynamic cine CMR, where the heart is imaged throughout the cardiac cycle, allowing AI to track the motion and deformation of the heart's chambers over time [70].

CNNs, a type of DL model, are particularly well-suited for image analysis tasks like segmentation. CNNs process input images hierarchically, detecting low-level features such as edges and gradients and progressively identifying more complex structures like the boundaries of the ventricles [71, 72]. By leveraging 3D CNNs, which account for spatial information across multiple slices, AI can produce precise volumetric assessments of the heart [73]. For example, AI systems can automate the calculation of end-diastolic volume (EDV)—the volume of blood in the ventricles at the end of diastole—and end-systolic volume (ESV)—the volume of blood remaining after contraction. By subtracting the ESV from EDV, AI systems can derive the stroke volume (SV), which quantifies the amount of blood ejected with each heartbeat. Moreover, the left ventricular ejection fraction (LVEF), a crucial clinical metric in diagnosing and managing DCM, can be calculated as the percentage of EDV ejected during systole [74].

Automating the segmentation and quantification of these critical parameters reduces the time and enhances the reproducibility of measurements across operators and institutions

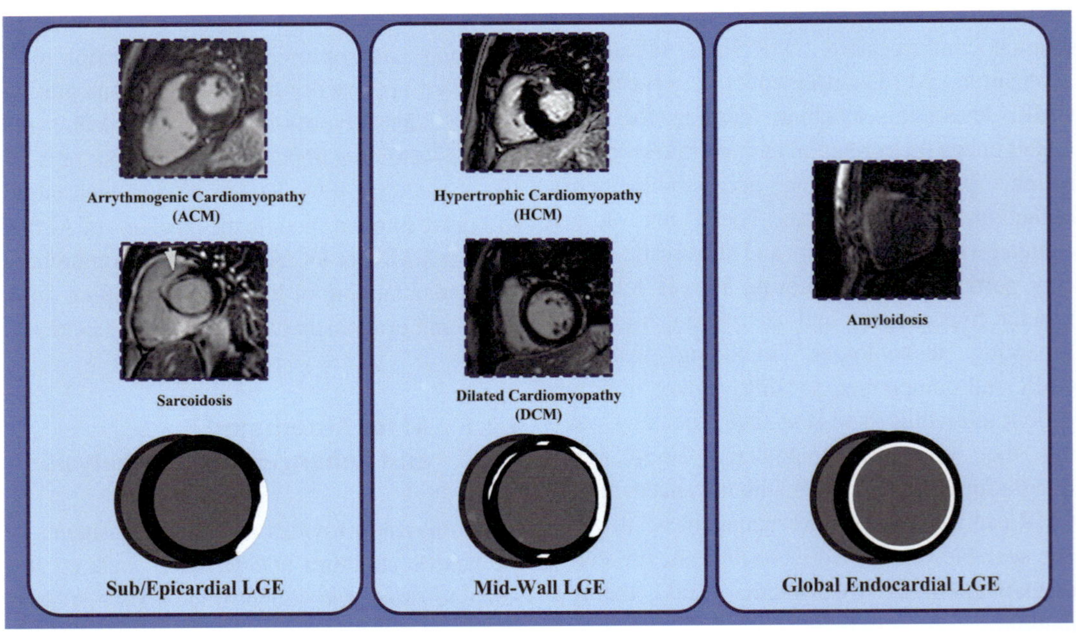

Fig. 3.1 Late gadolinium enhancement short axis images in different cardiomyopatheis

[75]. This is especially important in DCM, where even small changes in ventricular volumes or ejection fraction can significantly affect disease progression and treatment response. Early detection of declining ejection fraction in DCM patients can prompt timely therapeutic interventions, potentially delaying the onset of heart failure symptoms [76].

In addition to static measurements such as EDV and ESV, AI can unlock the full potential of cine CMR—a sequence of images taken throughout the cardiac cycle, capturing the heart's dynamic motion. Traditional CMR analysis often focuses on measurements at two discrete time points: end-diastole and end-systole. AI can analyze the entire cine loop, generating volume-time curves that reflect the variation in ventricular volumes throughout the cardiac cycle. This allows for the calculation of dynamic functional parameters, such as the peak ejection rate and the peak filling rate, which quantify the rates of blood ejection and ventricular filling, respectively [65, 77].

Dynamic functional parameters provide a more comprehensive picture of cardiac performance, capturing subtle systolic and diastolic function impairments. This is particularly valuable in DCM patients, where diastolic dysfunction—impaired ventricular filling—often coexists with systolic dysfunction—reduced ejection fraction. By automating the analysis of cine CMR, AI enables clinicians to detect early signs of functional impairment that may not be apparent through traditional metrics like LVEF alone [77, 78].

3.2.2 AI in Tissue Characterization: Detecting Fibrosis and Myocardial Changes

One of the most significant advantages of CMR is its ability to provide detailed information about myocardial tissue characteristics, particularly in detecting myocardial fibrosis. Fibrosis is a key marker of adverse remodeling in DCM and is associated with an increased risk of arrhythmias, heart failure, and sudden cardiac death [79]. CMR techniques such as late gadolinium enhancement (LGE) and T1 mapping allow for the non-invasive identification and quantification of both replacement fibrosis (scar tissue) and diffuse interstitial fibrosis [80].

LGE is a widely used CMR technique that highlights areas of replacement fibrosis by exploiting the differential uptake of gadolinium-based contrast agents. In DCM, mid-wall fibrosis is frequently observed, and its presence has been strongly linked to worse outcomes, including a higher risk of sudden cardiac death. Mid-wall fibrosis is a particularly important finding in DCM, as it differs from the subendocardial fibrosis typically seen in ischemic cardiomyopathy [50, 81].

AI, particularly U-Net architectures (a type of CNN specifically designed for segmentation), can automate the detection and quantification of fibrosis in LGE images. These models are trained to recognize patterns of gadolinium uptake that correspond to fibrotic tissue, allowing for precise and reproducible delineation of fibrotic regions. Once detected, AI can quantify the total fibrosis burden—typically expressed as a percentage of the total myocardial volume—providing clinicians with a robust measure of disease severity [82, 83].

Automating LGE analysis with AI systems reduces the subjectivity and inter-observer variability inherent in manual interpretation, ensuring that fibrosis assessments are consistent across institutions and operators [82]. This is particularly important for longitudinal monitoring of DCM patients, where changes in fibrosis burden over time can guide therapeutic decision-making [84].

While LGE is highly effective for detecting replacement fibrosis, it is less sensitive to diffuse interstitial fibrosis, which is more evenly distributed throughout the myocardium [80, 85]. Diffuse fibrosis results from the accumulation of extracellular matrix proteins in the interstitial space and is a hallmark of chronic myocardial remodeling. T1 mapping is a CMR technique that allows for the quantification of diffuse fibrosis by measuring the T1 relaxation time of myocardial tissue. Elevated T1 values are indicative of increased extracellular volume (ECV), which corresponds to the accumulation of fibrotic tissue [86].

AI can enhance the utility of T1 mapping by automating several critical steps in the analysis process. AI algorithms can perform motion correction and image registration, which are necessary for aligning pre-contrast and post-contrast images. This alignment is crucial for the accurate calculation of post-contrast T1 values and ECV. Once the images are aligned, AI can automate the calculation of extracellular volume (ECV).

Detecting early phases of diffuse fibrosis is particularly valuable in DCM patients, as it often precedes overt functional decline. Patients with preserved ejection fraction but elevated ECV are at increased risk of disease progression, arrhythmias, and heart failure [48, 80, 87, 88]. By identifying diffuse fibrosis before it leads to significant functional impairment, clinicians can intervene earlier, potentially delaying the onset of symptoms and improving long-term outcomes.

3.2.3 AI for Risk Stratification: Integrating Multi-dimensional Data

AI has the potential to revolutionize risk prediction by integrating a wide range of data types, including imaging biomarkers, clinical data, and genetic information. Imaging biomarkers such as fibrosis extent (from LGE) and extracellular volume (ECV) (from T1 mapping) can be combined with clinical parameters like age, comorbidities, and medication use to develop more comprehensive risk models [89–91]. Dynamic functional parameters, such as peak ejection and filling rates, can also be incorporated to provide a comprehensive assessment of cardiac function [77].

Moreover, AI can integrate genetic information into risk models to refine predictions. Certain genetic mutations, such as those in the LMNA and TTN genes, are associated with more aggressive forms of DCM and are linked to a higher likelihood of adverse outcomes [6, 92, 93]. By incorporating these genetic markers into the risk model, AI can help clinicians identify patients who may require closer monitoring or early intervention, even if their LVEF is not severely reduced.

For example, the *PLN p.Arg14del* mutation, which is associated with a higher risk of arrhythmias and fibrosis in DCM, can be integrated into AI-powered risk models [94]. AI can analyze the relationship between genetic mutations and specific imaging findings, such as fibrosis extent, to identify patients who may benefit from prophylactic ICD placement, even if they are not candidates for these procedures based on traditional criteria.

The ability of AI to integrate and analyze multi-dimensional data enables the creation of personalized risk models that reflect individual patients' unique clinical, genetic, and imaging profiles [95, 96]. This represents a significant shift towards precision medicine in DCM, where treatment decisions are tailored to the specific risk profile of each patient rather than relying on population-based thresholds such as LVEF alone.

AI is profoundly transforming the role of cardiac MRI (CMR) in the diagnosis, management, and risk stratification of dilated cardiomyopathy (DCM). By automating image analysis, AI enhances the precision, efficiency, and reproducibility of critical measurements such as ventricular volumes, ejection fraction, and myocardial mass. Beyond functional assessments, AI is instrumental in improving the detection and quantification of myocardial fibrosis, a key prognostic marker in DCM. Techniques such as late gadolinium enhancement (LGE) and T1 mapping benefit from AI-driven automation, allowing for more accurate and consistent tissue characterization.

Moreover, AI's ability to integrate multimodal data—including imaging biomarkers, clinical information, and genetic data—offers a more comprehensive and personalized approach for risk stratification. As AI technology continues to evolve, it will play an increasingly critical role in the management of DCM, offering new opportunities to improve patient outcomes through precision medicine.

3.3 Restrictive Cardiomyopathy (RCM): Overcoming Diagnostic Challenges

The presence of non-dilated left or right ventricular restrictive pathophysiology defines restrictive cardiomyopathy (RCM). This condition is accompanied by normal ventricular wall thickness and either normal or diminished diastolic and/or systolic volumes in one or both ventricles. Usually, systolic function remains intact until the disease reaches an advanced stage [97, 98].

RCM includes a range of diseases characterized by restricted left ventricular function. In RCM, the ventricular pressure increases quickly with minimal filling volume due to increased stiffness of the heart muscle. RCM is marked by long-term restrictive heart function, diastolic dysfunction, normal-sized ventricles, and enlarged atria, regardless of ventricular wall thickness and systolic function. Although RCM cases share common hemodynamic features, they can manifest in various ways.

Additionally, some patients may present with a combination of hypertrophic and restrictive phenotypes, making their classification challenging. Restrictive pathophysiology can be confirmed by cardiac catheterization or Doppler echocardiography. Diagnosis of specific conditions typically relies on clinical data, 12-lead electrocardiogram, echocardiography, nuclear medicine, or cardiovascular magnetic resonance imaging. Diagnosis may be challenging, as echocardiography, electrocardiograms, and lab tests can reveal non-specific changes. In such cases, cardiac magnetic resonance (CMR) could play an important role in diagnosis and treatment planning. CMR provides a detailed characterization of myocardial tissue based on the magnetic properties of abnormal areas, reducing the need for additional steps; however, further investigations, such as endomyocardial biopsy and genetic evaluation, may be necessary in certain cases [97].

CMR is an increasingly robust and noninvasive imaging technique for diagnosing various types of RCMs. Myocardial tissue characterization using advanced T1 and T2 mapping techniques can help identify storage or infiltrative conditions associated with specific changes in myocardial relaxation properties. These can also reveal diffuse inflammation or fibrosis in the myocardium [99–101].

New techniques using Artificial Intelligence (AI), machine learning (ML), and deep learning (DL) subsets [102–106] could provide more accurate classification and identification in patients with cardiomyopathy. These methods offer a potential solution to overcome the limitations associated with traditional approaches and improve personalized medicine [107].

Regarding Cardiac MR, non-contrast CMR examinations combined with AI have demonstrated promising results. They enable faster, more accessible, and cost-effective images, providing clear advantages in the clinical assessment of cardiomyopathies [26]. AI models can integrate various data types, such as demographic, clinical, genetic, ECG, echocardiography, CMR, and nuclear images, to comprehensively evaluate cardiomyopathy phenotypes [108].

The differentiation between RCM and constrictive pericarditis (CP) can be challenging due to similar clinical presentations and restrictive patterns presented with diastolic dysfunction [97].

Chao et al. utilized an apical four-chamber view in a transthoracic echocardiographic study to train a ResNet50 deep learning model. The model shows high reliability and an area under the curve of 0.97. It Effectively distinguishes between constrictive pericarditis and cardiac amyloidosis, making it a reliable diagnostic tool [109].

Additionally, Sengupta et al. have developed a machine-learning approach that integrates clinical parameters and conventional and speckle-tracking echocardiography (STE) data to differentiate between RCM and constrictive pericarditis. The associative memory classifier showed the best diagnostic performance, with an accuracy of 93.7% and an area under the curve of 96.2%. This study utilized a complicated chronic disease model of CP and RCM to show how a cognitive computing machine-learning approach could effectively automate interpretations of STE data. Integrating a cognitive computing machine-learning algorithm into cardiac imaging can help standardize assessments and improve the quality of interpretations, especially for readers with limited experience [110].

Another cardiac condition that may lead to a restrictive pattern is thalassemia. AI-based models have been developed to detect and measure iron deposits in the heart, helping in the early identification of myocardial dysfunction and timely intervention.

Taleie et al. developed a machine learning model to differentiate between beta-thalassemia major patients with and without myocardial iron overload, using radiomics features from echocardiographic images. The maximum relevance—minimum redundancy—and extreme gradient boosting model showed the best machine learning model results. An area under the curve (AUC) was 0.73, an accuracy of 0.73, a specificity of 0.73, and a sensitivity of 0.73. This shows that with non-invasive, cheap, and very accessible echocardiography, it is possible to determine who is prone to heart problems caused by iron overload in the future. It can lead to proper treatment to prevent heart problems and death [111]. Asmarian et al. proposed a machine learning model to evaluate cardiac iron overload. The model achieved an AUC of 0.68 (95% CI 0.60, 0.75). Among the three machine learning methods evaluated in this study, LR was found to be the most effective in predicting cardiac iron overload, while RF was the most effective method for predicting liver iron overload in patients with beta-thalassemia [112].

Fabry disease is another cause of RCM. Its clinical manifestations are heterogeneous and multisystemic, which can complicate the correct diagnosis. The use of an Artificial Intelligence-based approach to identify Fabry disease in patients is suggested. This approach includes the review of health record data from 4978 affected individuals and 1,000,000 healthy controls. The AI model was developed using a training cohort that included 75% of all patients selected randomly to create a statistical "phenotypic biomarker" for Fabry disease. Afterward, the authors evaluated the likelihood of Fabry disease in each patient within the testing cohort, which consisted of the remaining 25% of patients. This method showed strong analytical performance, achieving an area under the curve (AUC) of 0.82 [113].

Eckstein et al. have developed a supervised machine-learning model that includes various strain parameters from the right atrium, left atrium, and right ventricle, along with metrics of cardiac function, to detect cardiac amyloidosis. This model uses multiple machine learning classification algorithms, like k-nearest neighbor, linear and non-linear support vector machines (SVM), and decision trees. The non-linear SVM showed excellent performance, with an accuracy rate of 90.9% and an area under the curve (AUC) of 0.996, outperforming the other machine learning algorithms evaluated in their study [114].

3.4 Arrhythmogenic Cardiomyopathy (ACM): AI-Enhanced Risk Assessment

Arrhythmogenic Cardiomyopathy (ACM) is a hereditary cardiomyopathy usually inherited with an autosomal dominant pattern [115, 116]. ACM arises from the progressive substitution of ventricular myocardium with fibrofatty tissue, resulting in predisposition to fatal arrhythmias and sudden cardiac death [115, 116]. This cardiomyopathy was initially termed "Arrhythmogenic Right Ventricular Dysplasia/Cardiomyopathy (ARVCD)," as it was considered a cardiomyopathy predisposing affected patients to fatal arrhythmias and sudden cardiac death, particularly involving the Right Ventricle (RV) [116, 117]. It was established that ACM often involves both ventricles or could even solely affect the LV; thus, it is known as "Arrhythmogenic Cardiomyopathy (ACM)" nowadays [118, 119]. ACM is one of the most common arrhythmogenic cardiomyopathies among young patients presenting with sudden cardiac death, accounting for approximately one-fifth of sudden cardiac deaths before age 35 [118, 120]. The prevalence of ACM is reported to be 1 in 2000 to 5000; however, it has been suggested that this prevalence might even be as high as 1 in 1000, given its under-recognition [121].

Unlike other cardiomyopathies, ACM exhibits a wide range of clinical phenotypes, suggesting the presence of complicated interactions between genetic and epigenetic factors and environmental elements [6, 118]. Diagnosing ACM is a great challenge, for there is no single modality specific enough to diagnose ACM. Consequently, complex diagnostic criteria composed of multiple diagnostic information are used to diagnose ACM [121]. Initially, the Task Force Criteria (TFC) was proposed in 1994 to guide the diagnosis of ARVC. Despite high specificity, this criteria lacked sensitivity [122]. Subsequent efforts to deploy new technology and knowledge to enhance the sensitivity of the original TFC criteria while maintaining the specificity resulted in the revised TFC established in 2010 [122]. Ultimately, the Padua criteria were introduced in 2020, appending further tissue characterization and Electrocardiogram (ECG) features to enhance the diagnostic accuracy, and also considered biventricular and dominant-left ACM along with the dominant-right variants [123]. Given the complexity of the diagnostic criteria, the diagnosis of the ACM is laborious and prone to errors [124].

Increasing efforts have been made to develop a deep learning model to reduce human effort in ACM diagnosis and even reduce the subjective nature of some of the criteria [120, 125–127].

3.5 Electrocardiography

The ECG assessment as a part of the diagnostic criteria—depolarization and repolarization criteria—for ACM diagnosis could be subjective and prone to misdiagnosis, especially in the absence of an ACM expert [125]. Furthermore, similarities of other conditions—e.g., athletes' heart, dilated cardiomyopathy, cardiac sarcoidosis—might be difficult to discriminate, given their subtle differences [125, 128, 129]. Deep learning's clinical application for ECG interpretation is of increasing interest in the literature, and its application in ECG interpretation for ACM diagnosis is not an exception [125, 130].

The rarity of ACM could hinder training a deep learning model, which mandates large data sets to train well and overcome overfitting [131]. Preprocessing methods, such as data augmentation, could attenuate this shortcoming.

Haq et al. trained a Convolutional Neural Network to diagnose ACM using ECG [126]. ACM was diagnosed according to TFC 2010 in their study, and they did not utilize any data augmentation techniques to enhance their training set [126]. Their model achieved an Area Under the Curve (AUC) of 0.75 and 0.76 for rhythm and median beat ECG, respectively [126]. On the other hand, Carrick et al., after augmenting their data set, employed a neural network trained on ECG voltage tracings to discriminate ACM, diagnosed based on TFC 2010 [125]. The trained model attained excellent discrimination only using ECG to diagnose ACM (c-statistic 0.87 [0.86, 0.89]), which was comparable to ACM expert (0.85 [0.84, 0.86]) and surpassed non-ACM expert cardiologists (0.53 [CI: 0.52, 0.53]) [125]. Deep learning ECG interpreter enables an accurate and standard interpretation of the ECG to at least screen for ACM [125].

After conducting signal enhancement—omitting undesired noise from ECG paper traces—Papageorgiou et al. trained a low-complexity Convolutional Neural Network, achieving 98.6% accuracy in the detection of ACM within their test set [120]. The ECG and arrhythmia criteria are the most fruitful criteria for the first-line screening for the ACM [124]. An effective ECG screening—a low-cost and readily available modality—using deep learning models could theoretically prevent sudden cardiac death due to ARVC [120].

PLN *p.Arg14del* mutation is a risk factor for developing dilated or arrhythmogenic cardiomyopathy and is one of the diagnostic criteria of ACM [132]. Bleijendaal et al. employed and compared multiple machine learning and deep learning methods with experts in detecting the PLN *p.Arg14del* mutation from ECG. The experts outperformed all models regarding specificity; however, all machine learning and deep learning models surpassed experts regarding sensitivity, with the range for models 0.65 to 0.81 and that of experts 0.25 to 0.32 [132]. The overall accuracy of all models was superior to that of experts, with the highest accuracy being 0.76 for wavelet-machine learning-based models using logistic regression or support vector machine. These machine learning models outperformed deep learning models—i.e., convolutional neural networks and long short-term memory [132]. Currently, these models cannot be employed independently in the clinical setting; however, they could aid clinicians in enhancing their sensitivity and, thus, patient risk stratification.

3.6 Cardiac Magnetic Resonance Imaging

CMR is the best-suited modality for functional and structural evaluation and ACM tissue characterization [121]. CMR alone could provide one minor or two major scores according to TFC 2010, and the Padua criteria for right ventricle ACM [122, 123]. Thus, a precise assessment of the CMR is crucial [133]. The CMR segmentation—for measuring the indicated parameters for ACM diagnosis—is time-consuming and is prone to inter- and intra-observer variability, given that it is primarily based on RV, which is challenging to segment [133].

Misinterpretation of the CMR has been suggested to be the most common contributor to the misdiagnosis of the ACM [134]. Manual interpretation of the CMR is susceptible to bias and low reproducibility; therefore, attempts have been made to employ a deep learning model to standardize its interpretation and enhance reproducibility [127]. Isensee et al. trained a model to predict cardiac remodeling based on CMR. They preprocessed their dataset using resampling and normalization methods. A combination of modified 2D and 3D UNets was deployed to train the model for segmentation [127]. After that, instant features were extracted from the end-diastolic and end-systolic images. Subsequently, anatomical segmentation was conducted throughout the entire cardiac cycle, and dynamic features were measured and extracted accordingly [127]. Ultimately, 50 multilayer perceptrons (MLP) and a random forest were employed to classify pathologies [127]. They achieved an overall accuracy of 94% for cardiac pathology classification [127]. Another similar study also demonstrated that their deep learning CMR interpreter attains accuracy similar to that of human experts—96% correlation score—for cardiac pathology classification [135]. Although ACM was not among their classifications, the class of abnormal right ventricle determines that deep learning models could potentially be used to standardize the RV evaluation and ACM diagnosis.

Bourfiss et al. trained a deep learning model to interpret CMR for ACM diagnosis according to TFC 2010 [133]. After intensity normalization and data augmentation, they deployed the Bayesian Dilated Residual Neural Network to perform segmentation after training. Instant and dynamic features were extracted from segmented cine images [133]. Considering the basal region is the most susceptible region to segmentation inaccuracy, they repeated the classification model after correcting basal slice segmentation using expert annotations to evaluate the impact of basal segment inaccuracies on the overall results [133]. This correction of automated segmentation of the basal region resulted in enhanced segmentation in both end-diastolic and end-systolic slices for both ventricles [133].

While the neural network model slightly underestimated volume measures, the Ejection Fraction (EF) and Stroke Volume (SV) were somewhat overestimated by the model. Despite that, all measures estimated by the trained model had good to excellent correlation with that of the expert [133]. The basal region segmentation correction also enhances the accuracy of these measures—both volume and functional—to the extent to which they all attained excellent correlations [133]. Ultimately, classification of the patients using the model with basal segmentation correction classified all patients according to TFC 2010—i.e., no, minor, or major criteria—similar to manual labeling, except for one patient. One patient was classified as having minor criteria, while the manual labeling determined major criteria [133].

From a more pragmatic point of view, the deep learning model, although it performed well with a high correlation to the expert, the basal segment correction—which was human-based—played a crucial part [133]. Another study also observed this, suggesting that expert correction of deep learning model segmentation would enhance the accuracy of the classification model, determining cardiac pathology from CMR [136]. Utilizing deep learning models to aid the expert during the segmentation and interpretations could be more reliable and pragmatic than relying on the trained models to conduct fully automated segmentation and interpretation [133]. The semi-automated approach reduced the human effort and might, theoretically, reduce the inter- and intra-observer variability of CMR interpretation for ACM.

Strain parameters derived from feature-tracking CMR are gaining more recognition to aid earlier and enhanced diagnosis of ACM through earlier detection of subtle myocardial dysfunctions [119]. Along with global and regional strains exhibiting promising results in ACM diagnosis, novel strain parameters such as Longitudinal to Radial Strain Loop (LRSL) attained high accuracy [119]. Convolutional neural network exhibited encouraging accuracy in strain analysis in Hypertrophic cardiomyopathy patients [137]. Deep learning models also attained a high correlation to feature tracking for strain analysis of post-myocardial infarction patients [138].

Attempts have been made to develop a deep-learning model trained to conduct strain analysis in ACM. Alvarez-Florez et al. developed a deep learning model integrating information on CMR short-axis, long-axis, and four-chamber views [139]. They used Implicit Neural Representations to register CMR images, then conducted biomechanically informed regularization and enhanced resolution by deploying a super-resolution deep learning model [139]. They calculated radial and circumferential peak strain values after registration. ACM patients had significantly lower global radial strains in LV and RV compared to healthy controls [139]. It is proposed that the automated deep learning-based strain analysis might be beneficial for ACM diagnosis [139].

Employing a deep-learning model seems promising in ACM diagnosis, both for strain analysis from crude CMR cine images and for interpreting strains derived from feature tracking.

Detailed features of each type of cardiomyopathy are mentioned in Table 3.1 and Fig. 3.1.

Table 3.1 Comparison of DCM, HCM, ACM, and RCM in cardiac MRI and suggested features for deep learning models

Feature	Dilated Cardiomyopathy (DCM)	Hypertrophic Cardiomyopathy (HCM)	Arrhythmogenic Cardiomyopathy (ACM)	Restrictive Cardiomyopathy (RCM)
Chamber size	Dilated left or both ventricles; global enlargement	Asymmetrical or concentric hypertrophy, often septal predominance	Right ventricle (RV) dilation and thinning of the RV wall	Normal or small ventricles; biatrial enlargement
Wall thickness	Thin walls due to ventricular dilation	Thickened ventricular walls ($\geq$15 mm in HCM patients)	Focal thinning of the RV wall with fat or fibrosis infiltration	Normal wall thickness
Function	Decreased systolic function; reduced ejection fraction (EF)	Hyperdynamic LV function or localized LV outflow tract obstruction	RV dysfunction, occasionally LV involvement in advanced stages	Preserved EF, impaired diastolic function
Late gadolinium enhancement (LGE)	Linear mid-wall fibrosis in the septum or lateral walls	Patchy or diffuse LGE, often in hypertrophied areas or RV insertion points	Fibrofatty replacement predominantly in the RV; subepicardial fibrosis	Diffuse subendocardial fibrosis; non-coronary distribution

(continued)

Table 3.1 (continued)

Feature	Dilated Cardiomyopathy (DCM)	Hypertrophic Cardiomyopathy (HCM)	Arrhythmogenic Cardiomyopathy (ACM)	Restrictive Cardiomyopathy (RCM)
Cine imaging	Global hypokinesis, dilated chambers	Asymmetrical hypertrophy, LV outflow tract obstruction is visible in systole	RV akinesia, dyskinesia, or aneurysm formation	Restricted ventricular filling with normal chamber size and wall motion
T1/T2 mapping	Elevated native T1 and extracellular volume (ECV) due to fibrosis	Elevated T1 and ECV in fibrotic or hypertrophied regions	Elevated T1 and ECV in fibrotic areas; fatty infiltration lowers T1	Elevated T1 and ECV indicating diffuse fibrosis
Fatty infiltration	Not characteristic	Not characteristic	Common in RV walls and subepicardial LV regions	Not characteristic
Common symptoms	Heart failure, fatigue, dyspnea, arrhythmias	Syncope, exertional dyspnea, chest pain, arrhythmias, sudden death	Palpitations, arrhythmias, RV failure, sudden cardiac death (SCD)	Heart failure symptoms, diastolic dysfunction, and thromboembolic events
Primary diagnostic findings	Global ventricular dilation with reduced systolic function	Regional hypertrophy with LGE in hypertrophied segments	RV structural and functional abnormalities; fibrofatty infiltration	Biatrial enlargement, diastolic dysfunction, subendocardial LGE

References

1. Sandy J, Gonzalez A, Hilmer MJ. Alternative paths to college completion: effect of attending a 2-year school on the probability of completing a 4-year degree. Econ Educ Rev. 2006;25(5):463–71.
2. Khan MA, et al. Global epidemiology of ischemic heart disease: results from the global burden of disease study. Cureus. 2020;12(7)
3. Haq IU, et al. Artificial intelligence in cardiovascular medicine: current insights and future prospects. Vasc Health Risk Manag. 2022:517–28.
4. Siontis KC, et al. Artificial intelligence-enhanced electrocardiography in cardiovascular disease management. Nat Rev Cardiol. 2021;18(7):465–78.
5. Elliott PM, et al. 2014 ESC guidelines on diagnosis and management of hypertrophic cardiomyopathy. Polish Heart J (Kardiologia Polska). 2014;72(11):1054–126.
6. Jolfayi AG, et al. Exploring TTN variants as genetic insights into cardiomyopathy pathogenesis and potential emerging clues to molecular mechanisms in cardiomyopathies. Sci Rep. 2024;14(1):5313.
7. Maron BJ, Maron MS. Hypertrophic cardiomyopathy. Lancet. 2013;381(9862):242–55.
8. Geske JB, Ommen SR, Gersh BJ. Hypertrophic cardiomyopathy: clinical update. JACC: Heart Failure. 2018;6(5):364–75.
9. Fogel AL, Kvedar JC. Artificial intelligence powers digital medicine. NPJ Digit Med. 2018;1(1):5.
10. Malik P, Pathania M, Rathaur VK. Overview of artificial intelligence in medicine. J Family Med Prim Care. 2019;8(7):2328–31.
11. Huckleberry J, et al. Accuracy of non-ECG–gated computed tomography angiography of the chest in assessment of left-sided cardiac chamber enlargement. J Thorac Imaging. 2012;27(6):354–8.
12. Kathiria NN, et al. Assessment of left ventricular enlargement at multidetector computed tomography. J Comput Assist Tomogr. 2015;39(5):794–6.
13. Maron BJ, et al. Diagnosis and evaluation of hypertrophic cardiomyopathy: JACC state-of-the-art review. J Am Coll Cardiol. 2022;79(4):372–89.
14. Ommen SR, et al. 2020 AHA/ACC guideline for the diagnosis and treatment of patients with hypertrophic cardiomyopathy: a report of the American College of Cardiology/American Heart Association Joint Committee on Clinical Practice Guidelines. J Am Coll Cardiol. 2020;76(25):e159–240.
15. Olivotto I, et al. Assessment and significance of left ventricular mass by cardiovascular magnetic resonance in hypertrophic cardiomyopathy. J Am Coll Cardiol. 2008;52(7):559–66.
16. Amano Y, et al. Cardiac MR imaging of hypertrophic cardiomyopathy: techniques, findings, and clinical relevance. Magn Reson Med Sci. 2018;17(2):120–31.
17. Baggiano A, et al. Role of CMR mapping techniques in cardiac hypertrophic phenotype. Diagnostics. 2020;10(10):770.

18. Messroghli DR, et al. Clinical recommendations for cardiovascular magnetic resonance mapping of T1, T2, T2* and extracellular volume: a consensus statement by the Society for Cardiovascular Magnetic Resonance (SCMR) endorsed by the European Association for Cardiovascular Imaging (EACVI). J Cardiovasc Magn Reson. 2016;19(1):75.
19. Xu J, et al. MRI T1 mapping in hypertrophic cardiomyopathy: evaluation in patients without late gadolinium enhancement and hemodynamic obstruction. Radiology. 2020;294(2):275–86.
20. Dass S, et al. Myocardial tissue characterization using magnetic resonance noncontrast t1 mapping in hypertrophic and dilated cardiomyopathy. Circ Cardiovasc Imaging. 2012;5(6):726–33.
21. Lu M, et al. T1 mapping for detection of left ventricular myocardial fibrosis in hypertrophic cardiomyopathy: a preliminary study. Eur J Radiol. 2013;82(5):e225–31.
22. Bull S, et al. Human non-contrast T1 values and correlation with histology in diffuse fibrosis. Heart. 2013;99(13):932–7.
23. Bing R, Dweck MR. Myocardial fibrosis: why image, how to image and clinical implications. Heart. 2019;105(23):1832–40.
24. Diao K-Y, et al. Histologic validation of myocardial fibrosis measured by T1 mapping: a systematic review and meta-analysis. J Cardiovasc Magn Reson. 2017;18:1–11.
25. Schelbert EB, Messroghli DR. State of the art: clinical applications of cardiac T1 mapping. Radiology. 2016;278(3):658–76.
26. Cau R, et al. Artificial intelligence applications in cardiovascular magnetic resonance imaging: are we on the path to avoiding the administration of contrast media? Diagnostics. 2023;13(12):2061.
27. GhaffariJolfayi A, et al. Machine learning-based interpretation of non-contrast feature tracking strain analysis and T1/T2 mapping for assessing myocardial viability. Sci Rep. 2025;15(1):753.
28. Masoomi Z, et al. Prevalence of contrast-induced nephropathy after primary percutaneous coronary intervention at a tertiary referral hospital. Heliyon. 2024;10(4)
29. Zhang Q, et al. Artificial intelligence for contrast-free MRI: scar assessment in myocardial infarction using deep learning–based virtual native enhancement. Circulation. 2022;146(20):1492–503.
30. Zhang Q, et al. Toward replacing late gadolinium enhancement with artificial intelligence virtual native enhancement for gadolinium-free cardiovascular magnetic resonance tissue characterization in hypertrophic cardiomyopathy. Circulation. 2021;144(8):589–99.
31. Hansen MW, Merchant N. MRI of hypertrophic cardiomyopathy: part 2, differential diagnosis, risk stratification, and posttreatment MRI appearances. Am J Roentgenol. 2007;189(6):1344–52.
32. Mentias A, et al. Late gadolinium enhancement in patients with hypertrophic cardiomyopathy and preserved systolic function. J Am Coll Cardiol. 2018;72(8):857–70.
33. Kim RJ, et al. The use of contrast-enhanced magnetic resonance imaging to identify reversible myocardial dysfunction. N Engl J Med. 2000;343(20):1445–53.
34. Bruder O, et al. European cardiovascular magnetic resonance (EuroCMR) registry–multi national results from 57 centers in 15 countries. J Cardiovasc Magn Reson. 2013;15(1):9.
35. Mahrholdt H, et al. Delayed enhancement cardiovascular magnetic resonance assessment of non-ischaemic cardiomyopathies. Eur Heart J. 2005;26(15):1461–74.
36. Becker MA, et al. The prognostic value of late gadolinium-enhanced cardiac magnetic resonance imaging in nonischemic dilated cardiomyopathy: a review and meta-analysis. JACC Cardiovasc Imaging. 2018;11(9):1274–84.
37. Gerber BL, et al. Prognostic value of myocardial viability by delayed-enhanced magnetic resonance in patients with coronary artery disease and low ejection fraction: impact of revascularization therapy. J Am Coll Cardiol. 2012;59(9):825–35.
38. Gersh BJ, et al. 2011 ACCF/AHA guideline for the diagnosis and treatment of hypertrophic cardiomyopathy: executive summary: a report of the American College of Cardiology Foundation/American Heart Association Task Force on Practice Guidelines. Circulation. 2011;124(24):2761–96.
39. Burrage MK, Ferreira VM. Cardiovascular magnetic resonance for the differentiation of left ventricular hypertrophy. Curr Heart Fail Rep. 2020;17:192–204.
40. Muneretto C, et al. 2014 ESC guidelines on diagnosis and management of hypertrophic cardiomyopathy. Eur Heart J. 2014;35(39):2733–79.
41. Weng Z, et al. Prognostic value of LGE-CMR in HCM: a meta-analysis. JACC Cardiovasc Imaging. 2016;9(12):1392–402.
42. Ommen SR, et al. AHA/ACC guideline for the diagnosis and treatment of patients with hypertrophic cardiomyopathy a report of the American College of Cardiology/American Heart Association joint committee on clinical practice guidelines. Circulation. 2020;142(25):E558–631.
43. Kramer CM, et al. Hypertrophic cardiomyopathy registry: the rationale and design of an international, observational study of hypertrophic cardiomyopathy. Am Heart J. 2015;170(2):223–30.
44. Cowling T, Frey N. Macrocyclic and linear gadolinium based contrast agents for adults undergoing magnetic resonance imaging: a review of safety; 2019.
45. Oksuz I, et al. Deep learning using K-space based data augmentation for automated cardiac MR motion artefact detection. In: Medical image computing and computer assisted intervention–MICCAI 2018: 21st international conference, Granada, Spain, September 16–20, 2018, proceedings, part I. Springer; 2018.

46. Libby P. Braunwald's heart disease-E-book: a textbook of cardiovascular medicine. Elsevier Health Sciences; 2021.
47. Debus A, Ferrante E. Left ventricle quantification through spatio-temporal CNNs. In: Statistical atlases and computational models of the heart. atrial segmentation and LV quantification challenges: 9th international workshop, STACOM 2018, held in conjunction with MICCAI 2018, Granada, Spain, September 16, 2018, revised selected papers 9. Springer; 2019.
48. Vita T, et al. Comparing CMR mapping methods and myocardial patterns toward heart failure outcomes in nonischemic dilated cardiomyopathy. JACC Cardiovasc Imaging. 2019;12(8 Part 2):1659–69.
49. Charron P, et al. The cardiomyopathy registry of the EURObservational research Programme of the European Society of Cardiology: baseline data and contemporary management of adult patients with cardiomyopathies. Eur Heart J. 2018;39(20):1784–93.
50. Di Marco A, et al. Late gadolinium enhancement and the risk for ventricular arrhythmias or sudden death in dilated cardiomyopathy: systematic review and meta-analysis. JACC Heart Failure. 2017;5(1):28–38.
51. Guo J, et al. Artificial intelligence study on left ventricular function among normal individuals, hypertrophic cardiomyopathy and dilated cardiomyopathy patients using 1.5 T cardiac cine MR images obtained by SSFP sequence. Br J Radiol. 2022;95(1133):20201060.
52. Chen W-W, et al. A deep learning approach to classify fabry cardiomyopathy from hypertrophic cardiomyopathy using cine imaging on cardiac magnetic resonance. Int J Biomed Imaging. 2024;2024(1):6114826.
53. Hindieh W, et al. Discrepant measurements of maximal left ventricular wall thickness between cardiac magnetic resonance imaging and echocardiography in patients with hypertrophic cardiomyopathy. Circ Cardiovasc Imaging. 2017;10(8):e006309.
54. Sivalokanathan S, et al. Hypertrophic cardiomyopathy patients with paroxysmal atrial fibrillation have a high burden of left atrial fibrosis by cardiac magnetic resonance imaging. JACC Clin Electrophysiol. 2019;5(3):364–75.
55. Salmanipour A, et al. The predictive value of cardiac MRI strain parameters in hypertrophic cardiomyopathy patients with preserved left ventricular ejection fraction and a low fibrosis burden: a retrospective cohort study. Front Cardiovasc Med. 2023:10.
56. Ariga R, et al. Identification of myocardial disarray in patients with hypertrophic cardiomyopathy and ventricular arrhythmias. J Am Coll Cardiol. 2019;73(20):2493–502.
57. Neubauer S, et al. Distinct subgroups in hypertrophic cardiomyopathy in the NHLBI HCM registry. J Am Coll Cardiol. 2019;74(19):2333–45.
58. Marstrand P, et al. Hypertrophic cardiomyopathy with left ventricular systolic dysfunction: insights from the SHaRe registry. Circulation. 2020;141(17):1371–83.
59. Hirai K, et al. Feasibility of contrast-enhanced coronary artery magnetic resonance angiography using compressed sensing. J Cardiovasc Magn Reson. 2020;22(1):15.
60. Schukro C, Puchner SB. Safety and efficiency of low-field magnetic resonance imaging in patients with cardiac rhythm management devices. Eur J Radiol. 2019;118:96–100.
61. Simonetti OP, Ahmad R. Low-field cardiac magnetic resonance imaging: a compelling case for cardiac magnetic resonance's future. Circ Cardiovasc Imaging. 2017;10(6):e005446.
62. Weintraub RG, Semsarian C, Macdonald P. Dilated cardiomyopathy. Lancet. 2017;390(10092):400–14.
63. Halliday BP, et al. Personalizing risk stratification for sudden death in dilated cardiomyopathy: the past, present, and future. Circulation. 2017;136(2):215–31.
64. Francone M. Role of cardiac magnetic resonance in the evaluation of dilated cardiomyopathy: diagnostic contribution and prognostic significance. Int Schol Res Notices. 2014;2014(1):365404.
65. Asher C, et al. The role of AI in characterizing the DCM phenotype. Front. Cardiovasc Med. 2021;8:787614.
66. Johnson KB, et al. Precision medicine, AI, and the future of personalized health care. Clin Transl Sci. 2021;14(1):86–93.
67. Kramer CM, et al. Standardized cardiovascular magnetic resonance imaging (CMR) protocols, society for cardiovascular magnetic resonance: board of trustees task force on standardized protocols. J Cardiovasc Magn Reson. 2008;10:1–10.
68. Suinesiaputra A, et al. Quantification of LV function and mass by cardiovascular magnetic resonance: multi-center variability and consensus contours. J Cardiovasc Magn Reson. 2015;17:1–8.
69. Yasaka K, et al. Deep learning with convolutional neural network in radiology. Jpn J Radiol. 2018;36:257–72.
70. Mariscal-Harana J, et al. An artificial intelligence tool for automated analysis of large-scale unstructured clinical cine cardiac magnetic resonance databases. Eur Heart J Digit Health. 2023;4(5):370–83.
71. Chen C, et al. Deep learning for cardiac image segmentation: a review. Front Cardiovasc Med. 2020;7:25.
72. Bai W, et al. Automated cardiovascular magnetic resonance image analysis with fully convolutional networks. J Cardiovasc Magn Reson. 2018;20(1):65.
73. Inomata S, et al. Estimation of left and right ventricular ejection fractions from cine-MRI using 3D-CNN. Sensors. 2023;23(14):6580.
74. Michler K, et al. Cardiac MRI: an alternative method to determine the left ventricular function. Diagnostics. 2023;13(8):1437.
75. Jafari M, et al. Automated diagnosis of cardiovascular diseases from cardiac magnetic resonance imag-

ing using deep learning models: a review. Comput Biol Med. 2023;160:106998.
76. Japp AG, et al. The diagnosis and evaluation of dilated cardiomyopathy. J Am Coll Cardiol. 2016;67(25):2996–3010.
77. Ruijsink B, et al. Fully automated, quality-controlled cardiac analysis from CMR: validation and large-scale application to characterize cardiac function. Cardiovasc Imaging. 2020;13(3):684–95.
78. Goyal N, et al. Machine learning based quantification of ejection and filling parameters by fully automated dynamic measurement of left ventricular volumes from cardiac magnetic resonance images. Magn Reson Imaging. 2020;67:28–32.
79. Assomull RG, et al. Cardiovascular magnetic resonance, fibrosis, and prognosis in dilated cardiomyopathy. J Am Coll Cardiol. 2006;48(10):1977–85.
80. aus dem Siepen F, et al. T1 mapping in dilated cardiomyopathy with cardiac magnetic resonance: quantification of diffuse myocardial fibrosis and comparison with endomyocardial biopsy. Eur Heart J Cardiovasc Imaging. 2015;16(2):210–6.
81. McCrohon J, et al. Differentiation of heart failure related to dilated cardiomyopathy and coronary artery disease using gadolinium-enhanced cardiovascular magnetic resonance. Circulation. 2003;108(1):54–9.
82. Zabihollahy F, Rajan S, Ukwatta E. Machine learning-based segmentation of left ventricular myocardial fibrosis from magnetic resonance imaging. Curr Cardiol Rep. 2020;22(8):65.
83. Fahmy AS, et al. Automated cardiac MR scar quantification in hypertrophic cardiomyopathy using deep convolutional neural networks. JACC Cardiovasc Imaging. 2018;11(12):1917–8.
84. Romano S, et al. Feature-tracking global longitudinal strain predicts death in a multicenter population of patients with ischemic and nonischemic dilated cardiomyopathy incremental to ejection fraction and late gadolinium enhancement. JACC Cardiovasc Imaging. 2018;11(10):1419–29.
85. Mewton N, et al. Assessment of myocardial fibrosis with cardiovascular magnetic resonance. J Am Coll Cardiol. 2011;57(8):891–903.
86. Haaf P, et al. Cardiac T1 mapping and extracellular volume (ECV) in clinical practice: a comprehensive review. J Cardiovasc Magn Reson. 2016;18(1):89.
87. Puntmann VO, et al. T1-mapping and outcome in nonischemic cardiomyopathy: all-cause mortality and heart failure. JACC Cardiovasc Imaging. 2016;9(1):40–50.
88. Barison A, et al. Prognostic significance of myocardial extracellular volume fraction in nonischaemic dilated cardiomyopathy. J Cardiovasc Med. 2015;16(10):681.
89. Faizal ASM, et al. A review of risk prediction models in cardiovascular disease: conventional approach vs. artificial intelligent approach. Comput Methods Prog Biomed. 2021;207:106190.
90. Juarez-Orozco LE, et al. Artificial intelligence to improve risk prediction with nuclear cardiac studies. Curr Cardiol Rep. 2022;24(4):307–16.
91. Stamate E, et al. Revolutionizing cardiology through artificial intelligence—big data from proactive prevention to precise diagnostics and cutting-edge treatment—a comprehensive review of the past 5 years. Diagnostics. 2024;14(11):1103.
92. Herman DS, et al. Truncations of titin causing dilated cardiomyopathy. N Engl J Med. 2012;366(7):619–28.
93. Glöcklhofer CR, et al. A novel LMNA nonsense mutation causes two distinct phenotypes of cardiomyopathy with high risk of sudden cardiac death in a large five-generation family. Ep Europace. 2018;20(12):2003–13.
94. Te Rijdt WP, et al. Myocardial fibrosis as an early feature in phospholamban p. Arg14del mutation carriers: phenotypic insights from cardiovascular magnetic resonance imaging. Euro Heart J Cardiovasc Imaging. 2019;20(1):92–100.
95. Singh M, et al. Artificial intelligence for cardiovascular disease risk assessment in personalised framework: a scoping review. EClinicalMedicine. 2024:73.
96. Haq I-U, Haq I, Xu B. Artificial intelligence in personalized cardiovascular medicine and cardiovascular imaging. Cardiovasc Diagn Ther. 2021;11(3):911.
97. Rapezzi C, et al. Restrictive cardiomyopathy: definition and diagnosis. Eur Heart J. 2022;43(45):4679–93.
98. Cimiotti D, et al. Genetic restrictive cardiomyopathy: causes and consequences—an integrative approach. Int J Mol Sci. 2021;22(2):558.
99. Galea N, et al. Cardiovascular magnetic resonance (CMR) in restrictive cardiomyopathies. Radiol Med. 2020;125:1072–86.
100. Chalian H, et al. The role of cardiac magnetic resonance imaging parameters in prognostication of systemic sclerosis in patients with cardiac involvement: a systematic review of the literature. Acad Radiol. 2024;
101. Ghaffari Jolfayi A, et al. Imaging findings in cardiovascular involvements of IgG4-related disease: a systematic review study. Rheumatology. 2024;
102. Cau R, et al. Long-COVID diagnosis: From diagnostic to advanced AI-driven models. Eur J Radiol. 2022;148:110164.
103. Cau R, et al. Potential role of artificial intelligence in cardiac magnetic resonance imaging: can it help clinicians in making a diagnosis? J Thorac Imaging. 2021;36(3):142–8.
104. Cau R, et al. Artificial intelligence in computed tomography plaque characterization: a review. Eur J Radiol. 2021;140:109767.
105. Dey D, et al. Artificial intelligence in cardiovascular imaging: JACC state-of-the-art review. J Am Coll Cardiol. 2019;73(11):1317–35.

106. Tang A, et al. Canadian Association of Radiologists white paper on artificial intelligence in radiology. Can Assoc Radiol J. 2018;69(2):120–35.
107. Kim K-H, et al. Artificial intelligence applied to cardiomyopathies: is it time for clinical application? Curr Cardiol Rep. 2022;24(11):1547–55.
108. Cau R, et al. Artificial intelligence in the differential diagnosis of cardiomyopathy phenotypes. Diagnostics. 2024;14(2):156.
109. Chao C-J, et al. Echocardiography-based deep learning model to differentiate constrictive pericarditis and restrictive cardiomyopathy. Cardiovasc Imaging. 2024;17(4):349–60.
110. Sengupta P, et al. Cognitive machine-learning algorithm for cardiac imaging: a pilot study for differentiating constrictive pericarditis from restrictive cardiomyopathy. Circ Cardiovasc Imaging. 2016;9:e004330. The first study to evaluate the role of automated machine-learning algorithms in differential diagnosis of constrictive pericarditis and restrictive cardiomyopathy
111. Taleie H, et al. Left ventricular myocardial dysfunction evaluation in thalassemia patients using echocardiographic radiomic features and machine learning algorithms. J Digit Imaging. 2023;36(6):2494–506.
112. Asmarian N, et al. Prediction of heart and liver iron overload in β-thalassemia major patients using machine learning methods. Hemoglobin. 2022;46(6):303–7.
113. Jefferies JL, et al. A new approach to identifying patients with elevated risk for Fabry disease using a machine learning algorithm. Orphanet J Rare Dis. 2021;16:1–8.
114. Eckstein J, et al. A machine learning challenge: detection of cardiac amyloidosis based on bi-atrial and right ventricular strain and cardiac function. Diagnostics. 2022;12(11):2693.
115. Azimi A, et al. Arrhythmogenic left ventricular cardiomyopathy caused by a novel likely pathogenic DSP mutation, p.K1165Rfs*8, in a family with sudden cardiac death. BMC Med Genom. 2023;16(1):266.
116. Miles C, et al. Sudden death and left ventricular involvement in Arrhythmogenic cardiomyopathy. Circulation. 2019;139(15):1786–97.
117. Corrado D, Basso C. Arrhythmogenic left ventricular cardiomyopathy. Heart. 2022;108(9):733–43.
118. Saffitz JE. Arrhythmogenic cardiomyopathy. Circulation. 2011;124(15):e390–2.
119. MozafaryBazargany M, et al. Value of cardiac magnetic resonance feature-tracking in Arrhythmogenic cardiomyopathy (ACM): a systematic review and meta-analysis. IJC Heart Vasc. 2024;53:101455.
120. Papageorgiou VE, et al. Analysis of digitalized ECG signals based on artificial intelligence and spectral analysis methods specialized in ARVC. Int J Numer Method Biomed Eng. 2022;38(11):e3644.
121. te Riele ASJM, Tandri H, Bluemke DA. Arrhythmogenic right ventricular cardiomyopathy (ARVC): cardiovascular magnetic resonance update. J Cardiovasc Magn Reson. 2014;16(1):50.
122. Marcus FI, et al. Diagnosis of Arrhythmogenic right ventricular cardiomyopathy/dysplasia. Circulation. 2010;121(13):1533–41.
123. Corrado D, et al. Diagnosis of arrhythmogenic cardiomyopathy: the Padua criteria. Int J Cardiol. 2020;319:106–14.
124. Bosman LP, et al. Diagnosing arrhythmogenic right ventricular cardiomyopathy by 2010 task force criteria: clinical performance and simplified practical implementation. EP Europace. 2020;22(5):787–96.
125. Carrick RT, et al. Improved diagnosis of arrhythmogenic right ventricular cardiomyopathy using electrocardiographic deep-learning. Heart Rhythm. 2024;
126. Haq IU, et al. Artificial intelligence-enhanced electrocardiogram for arrhythmogenic right ventricular cardiomyopathy detection. Eur Heart J Digit Health. 2024;5(2):192–4.
127. Isensee F, et al. Automatic cardiac disease assessment on cine-MRI via time-series segmentation and domain specific features. In: Statistical atlases and computational models of the heart. ACDC and MMWHS challenges: 8th international workshop, STACOM 2017, held in conjunction with MICCAI 2017, Quebec City, Canada, September 10-14, 2017, revised selected papers 8. Springer; 2018.
128. Philips B, et al. Arrhythmogenic right ventricular dysplasia/cardiomyopathy and cardiac sarcoidosis: distinguishing features when the diagnosis is unclear. Circ Arrhythm Electrophysiol. 2014;7(2):230–6.
129. Zaidi A, et al. Clinical differentiation between physiological remodeling and arrhythmogenic right ventricular cardiomyopathy in athletes with marked electrocardiographic repolarization anomalies. J Am Coll Cardiol. 2015;65(25):2702–11.
130. Avula V, Wu Katherine C, Carrick Richard T. Clinical applications, methodology, and scientific reporting of electrocardiogram deep-learning models. JACC Adv. 2023;2(10):100686.
131. Jiménez-Serrano S, et al. New ECG biomarkers and sex-stratified models for the detection of arrhythmogenic cardiomyopathy with left ventricular involvement. Available at SSRN 4824608.
132. Bleijendaal H, et al. Computer versus cardiologist: is a machine learning algorithm able to outperform an expert in diagnosing a phospholamban p.Arg14del mutation on the electrocardiogram? Heart Rhythm. 2021;18(1):79–87.
133. Bourfiss M, et al. Towards automatic classification of cardiovascular magnetic resonance task force criteria for diagnosis of arrhythmogenic right ventricular cardiomyopathy. Clin Res Cardiol. 2023;112(3):363–78.

134. Sampognaro JR, et al. Diagnostic pitfalls in patients referred for arrhythmogenic right ventricular cardiomyopathy. Heart Rhythm. 2023;20(12):1720–6.
135. Bernard O, et al. Deep learning techniques for automatic MRI cardiac multi-structures segmentation and diagnosis: is the problem solved? IEEE Trans Med Imaging. 2018;37(11):2514–25.
136. Huellebrand M, et al. A collaborative approach for the development and application of machine learning solutions for CMR-based cardiac disease classification. Front Cardiovasc Med. 2022:9.
137. Vigneault DM, et al. Feature tracking cardiac magnetic resonance via deep learning and spline optimization. In: Functional imaging and modelling of the heart. Cham: Springer; 2017.
138. Urmeneta Ulloa J, et al. Comparative cardiac magnetic resonance-based feature tracking and deep-learning strain assessment in patients hospitalized for acute myocarditis. J Clin Med. 2023;12 https://doi.org/10.3390/jcm12031113.
139. Alvarez-Florez L, et al. Deep learning for automatic strain quantification in arrhythmogenic right ventricular cardiomyopathy. In: International workshop on statistical atlases and computational models of the heart. Springer; 2023.

4 Coronary Artery Disease: Integration of Artificial Intelligence with Advanced Imaging Techniques for Detection and Management

Amir Ghaffari Jolfayi, Reza Elahi, Amir Azimi, Hosein Tanha, Saba Mehrtabar, Samin Sadraei, Shahrzad Shahrokhi Nejad, and Sanaz Asadian

Abstract

Coronary artery disease (CAD) remains a leading global cause of mortality, highlighting the need for innovative diagnostic and prognostic tools. Cardiac magnetic resonance (CMR), utilizing techniques such as stress perfusion imaging, late gadolinium enhancement (LGE), and T1/T2 mapping, provides unparalleled precision in assessing myocardial perfusion, viability, and structural abnormalities. On the other hand, Artificial Intelligence (AI) has revolutionized CAD diagnostics by employing machine learning (ML) and deep learning (DL) algorithms to automate and enhance interpretations of imaging modalities, including CMR, single-photon emission computed tomography (SPECT), positron emission tomography (PET), and coronary computed tomographic angiography (CCTA). These algorithms improve myocardial perfusion quantification, coronary artery calcification (CAC) scoring, and stenosis detection, addressing challenges such as clinician workload and inter-reader variability. Previous studies highlighted AI's ability to surpass traditional diagnostic methods, with tools like convolutional neural networks (CNNs), with acceptable sensitivity, specificity, and accuracy. The integration of CMR and AI represents a major advancement in non-invasive CAD management, enabling early detection, personalized treatment planning, and robust long-term prognostic evaluation.

Authors Amir Ghaffari Jolfayi and Reza Elahi have contributed equality and shared the first co-authorship.

A. Ghaffari Jolfayi · A. Azimi
Cardiovascular Imaging Research Center, Rajaie Cardiovascular Institute, Iran University of Medical Sciences, Tehran, Iran

R. Elahi
Department of Radiology, Zanjan University of Medical Sciences, Zanjan, Iran

H. Tanha
Clinical Research Development Unit, Mashhad University of Medical Sciences, Mashhad, Iran

S. Mehrtabar
Department of Radiology, Tabriz University of Medical Sciences, Tabriz, Iran

S. Sadraei · S. Shahrokhi Nejad
School of Medicine, Shahid Beheshti University of Medical Sciences, Tehran, Iran

S. Asadian (✉)
Department of Radiology, Cardiothoracic Imaging, University of Washington, Seattle, USA

A. Ghaffari Jolfayi (ed.), *Navigating Cardiology's Future*,
https://doi.org/10.1007/978-981-95-0313-1_4

By combining the detailed imaging capabilities of CMR with AI's analytical precision, this approach simplifies clinical workflows and reduces diagnostic uncertainty. These advancements highlight the potential of AI-enhanced imaging in transforming cardiovascular medicine.

This chapter focuses on the integration of AI with Imaging modalities, particularly advanced CMR techniques, to improve the detection, characterization, and management of CAD.

Keywords

Coronary artery disease · Cardiac magnetic resonance imaging · Artificial intelligence · Machine learning · Deep learning

Abbreviations

ACS	Acute Coronary Syndrome
AI	Artificial Intelligence.
ANNs	Artificial Neural Networks.
AUC	Area Under the Curve.
AUROC	Area Under the Receiver Operating Curve.
CAC	Coronary Artery Calcification.
CAD	Coronary Artery Disease.
CCTA	Coronary Computed Tomographic Angiography.
CMR	Cardiac Magnetic Resonance.
CNNs	Convolutional Neural Networks.
CT	Computed Tomography.
CVD	Cardiovascular Disease.
DL	Deep Learning.
ECG	Electrocardiogram.
eGFR	Estimated Glomerular Filtration Rate.
FFR	Fractional Flow Reserve.
FSE	Fast Spin-Echo.
GANs	Generative Adversarial Networks.
GBCAs	Gadolinium-based Contrast Agents.
LGE	Late Gadolinium Enhancement.
MI	Myocardial Infarction.
MINOCA	Myocardial Infarction with Non-Obstructive Coronary Arteries.
ML	Machine Learning.
MPI	Myocardial Perfusion Imaging.
MPS	Myocardial Perfusion Scintigraphy.
MRA	Magnetic Resonance Angiography.
MRI	Magnetic Resonance Imaging.
NSF	Nephrogenic Systemic Fibrosis.
PCI	Percutaneous Coronary Intervention.
PET	Positron Emission Tomography.
PSIR	Phase-Sensitive Inversion Recovery.
RF	Random Forest.
SPECT	Single-Photon Emission Computed Tomography.
SSFP	Steady-State Free Precession.
STEMI	ST-segment Elevation Myocardial Infarction.
STIR	Short T1 Inversion Recovery.
SVM	Support Vector Machine.
TPD	Total Perfusion Deficit.
XGBoost	eXtreme Gradient Boosting.
3D	Three-dimensional.

4.1 The Role of MRI in Detecting Coronary Artery Disease

Coronary artery disease (CAD) remains a leading cause of mortality globally, with its prevalence steadily rising [1, 2]. Various imaging techniques have been developed and employed to diagnose and assess the severity of CAD accurately [3, 4]. Magnetic resonance imaging (MRI) is one of the most precise and helpful imaging techniques. Both anatomical and functional aspects of the heart can be evaluated with cardiac MRI without ionizing radiation, compared with computed tomography (CT). Moreover, given its high tissue contrast and spatial resolution, cardiac MRI is preferred for evaluating myocardial perfusion, viability, and detecting ischemia. However, its application is limited by being time-consuming, expensive, and less widely available, as well as in claustrophobic patients or those with non-MRI-compatible implants.

4.1.1 Principles of Cardiac MRI

MRI relies on detecting signals generated by the abundant hydrogen nuclei in the human body [5]. When a patient is placed within a magnetic field (designated as B_0), the hydrogen nuclei align with this field, either parallel or antiparallel to the direction of B_0. The collective magnetic effect of these hydrogen nuclei is termed equilibrium magnetization, which can be excited by a radiofrequency (RF) pulse to produce an MRI signal [6].

Hydrogen nuclei in various tissue types (e.g., fat, proteins, fluids) resonate at distinct frequencies. Considering the resonance phenomenon, RF pulses are engineered to match the specific frequency of the hydrogen nuclei in different tissues, thereby generating a measurable signal that is characteristic of each tissue type. Spatial localization of hydrogen nuclei within the scanner is achieved using three-dimensional (3D) magnetic field gradients [7].

Following the application of an RF pulse, the absorbed electromagnetic energy is emitted back into the environment through two mechanisms: longitudinal magnetization recovery and transverse magnetization decay, quantified by the T1 and T2 (or T2*) relaxation times, respectively. These relaxation times allow MRI to utilize various pulse sequences to capture changes in these rates, thereby generating contrast in images to distinguish tissue types, differentiate between normal and pathological states, and assess the severity of tissue abnormalities [8].

The physiopathological characteristics of the examined tissue influence the choice of imaging technique and are the basis of signal contrast weighting. T1-weighted imaging is generally preferred for qualitative analysis, making T1-weighted pulse sequences the most commonly used in cardiac magnetic resonance (CMR). Typical T1-weighted CMR techniques include gradient echo cine imaging, myocardial perfusion imaging, late gadolinium enhancement (LGE), and phase contrast blood flow imaging. Conversely, T2-weighted and T2*-weighted CMR are primarily utilized for assessing myocardial edema and iron content, respectively. The cine steady-state free precession (SSFP) sequence, which provides a mixed T1/T2 weighting, is the standard method for evaluating cardiac volumes and functions [5].

4.1.2 Contrast Agents in CMR

Gadolinium-based contrast agents (GBCAs) are used in CMR [9]. After intravenous administration, a GBCA circulates through the cardiac chambers and coronary arteries for approximately 15–30 s during the first-pass phase before diffusing into the extracellular space. About 10–15 min later, a transient equilibrium is reached between the contrast agent accumulating in the extracellular space and its return to the blood pool. Currently, myocardial perfusion CMR and most magnetic resonance angiography (MRA) studies are conducted during the first-pass phase, while LGE imaging is performed during the equilibrium phase [10].

All GBCAs are chelated to prevent toxicity and facilitate renal excretion. While the use of GBCAs is generally associated with mild reactions, such as nausea and minor skin rashes, in approximately 1% of patients, severe reactions are exceedingly rare. However, in individuals with severe renal impairment, GBCA administration poses a risk of exposure to toxic, non-chelated gadolinium ions (Gd^{3+}), which can result in nephrogenic systemic fibrosis (NSF). NSF is an interstitial inflammatory condition that may lead to severe skin thickening, contractures, internal organ fibrosis, and even death. Risk factors for developing NSF include a low estimated glomerular filtration rate (eGFR), the need for hemodialysis, acute renal failure, and concurrent proinflammatory conditions [11].

Recent advancements to mitigate the risk of NSF include routine screening of at-risk patients using creatinine clearance assessments, weight-based dosing adjustments, avoiding GBCA use in patients with an eGFR below 30, and employing macrocyclic GBCAs. Over the past decade, these measures have led to a near-zero incidence of NSF globally. As of April 2020, the American College of Radiology has deemed the risk of NSF from macrocyclic GBCAs sufficiently low, potentially eliminating the need for routine questionnaire screening and eGFR testing in some cases [5].

4.1.3 CMR Imaging Methods

CMR imaging employs synchronization with the electrocardiogram (ECG) signal, known as cardiac gating, to mitigate the effects of cardiac motion blur. This gating can be either prospective, where ECG triggering occurs in real-time with image acquisition during each cardiac cycle, or retrospective, involving continuous data acquisition followed by reconstruction based on ECG timing. Retrospective gating is preferred for cine imaging due to its ability to cover the entire cardiac cycle comprehensively.

Several techniques are utilized to address blurring caused by respiratory motion. These include patient breath-holding, tracking diaphragmatic position and motion using navigator methods, and averaging respiratory motion. For patients unable to hold their breath or with irregular heart rhythms, static single-shot and real-time cine imaging—both involving rapid acquisition of whole images within a single cardiac cycle—can be employed, albeit at reduced temporal and spatial resolutions [12].

CMR utilizes both bright-blood cine SSFP imaging and dark-blood fast spin-echo (FSE) imaging to evaluate cardiac morphology and structure. Cine SSFP provides high temporal resolution imaging of the heart in motion, typically at 30 to 45 milliseconds per frame during a breath-hold of less than 10 s. For dark-blood imaging, T1-weighted FSE is used to visualize cardiac chambers, vascular structures, the pericardium, and fat. T2-weighted FSE with fat suppression is employed to assess myocardial edema [13].

Myocardial tagging, which involves marking the myocardium with dark lines or a grid to measure deformation across the cardiac cycle, has been extensively validated for assessing myocardial strain [14]. This technique quantifies global and regional myocardial performance in *circumferential*, *longitudinal*, and *radial* directions. However, the significant postprocessing requirements limit its clinical efficiency.

Feature tracking, which detects and follows the pattern of myocardial pixels at the blood pool-myocardial border across successive time frames, has gained clinical traction due to its application on routine cine SSFP imaging.

LGE is a T1-weighted imaging method that identifies GBCA accumulation in the myocardium due to infarction, infiltration, or fibrosis. LGE imaging, performed 5–15 min after GBCA injection (0.1–0.2 mmol/kg), can be captured in either 2D or 3D formats. Phase-sensitive inversion recovery (PSIR) reconstruction is routinely used to enhance myocardial tissue contrast in LGE imaging [15]. For patients unable to hold their breath, LGE imaging can be acquired using single-shot methods or navigator guidance.

The goal of CMR perfusion imaging is to track the first-pass transit of the GBCA bolus through the coronary circulation. Fast bright-blood gradient-echo imaging in three to five short-axis slices during each cardiac cycle is taken. In this way, a strong signal enhancement in well-perfused regions compared to hypo-enhancement in poorly perfused myocardium will be established [16].

T2-weighted imaging detects myocardial edema caused by ischemic injury or inflammation, strongly correlating with the area at risk following acute myocardial infarction (MI). It complements LGE in assessing MI chronicity and measuring salvageable myocardium. The pulse sequence options for T2-weighted imaging include black-blood short tau inversion recovery (STIR) FSE and newer SSFP-type methods.

$T2^*$ imaging, a well-validated method for measuring tissue iron content, identifies myocardial iron overload. A $T2^*$ of less than 20 milliseconds indicates iron overload, with values below 10 milliseconds suggesting severe iron overload. Despite challenges such as small luminal sizes and cardiac and respiratory motion artifacts, advances in coronary MRA imaging favor the use of whole-heart 3D acquisition (with or without navigator guidance) [17]. Phase contrast imaging quantifies blood flow velocities, myocardial motion, and intravascular flow rates.

MRI data acquisition is time-consuming, typically taking around 200 milliseconds to construct a single image. Parallel imaging techniques, which leverage the spatial coverage of phased-array surface coils, reduce the number of lines of raw data needed by two- to threefold [18]. These methods are routinely used in commercial MRI systems to decrease acquisition time and/or improve temporal resolution. Additionally, k-t accelerated imaging methods, which reconstruct images from a reduced amount of data based on temporal correlations, are now routinely employed in clinical practice.

4.1.4 Clinical Application of CMR in CAD

4.1.4.1 Stable Chest Pain Assessment

Recent evidence highlights the accuracy of vasodilating stress CMR perfusion imaging in diagnosing and risk-stratifying patients with stable chest pain syndromes. Stress CMR perfusion imaging offers several advantages over traditional methods, including reduced artifacts, absence of ionizing radiation, and threefold higher spatial resolution compared to single-photon emission computed tomography (SPECT). Studies have demonstrated that stress CMR perfusion is highly effective in detecting both single-vessel and multi-vessel CAD, outperforming SPECT in diagnostic accuracy.

The physiological assessment provided by stress CMR complements the evaluation of coronary atherosclerosis through calcium scoring [19]. Patients with a negative stress CMR consistently exhibit low annual cardiac event rates, as shown by numerous single and multicenter studies [20, 21]. For instance, a recent multicenter registry study involving 2349 patients found that those with a negative stress CMR had an annual cardiac event rate of only 0.6% over a 5-year follow-up period [22]. Stress CMR has also been shown to be cost-effective in this context [23].

Quantitative stress CMR perfusion, utilizing automated algorithms, is increasingly becoming the standard of care in some experienced CMR centers. This approach offers potential advantages over qualitative methods, including reduced reader bias, improved assessment of microvascular coronary disease, and enhanced diagnostic accuracy, particularly in cases of possible multi-vessel CAD [24] and prognostication of adverse cardiac events [25]. Previous investigations have confirmed the high correlation between stress CMR perfusion and invasive fractional flow reserve (FFR) measurements, underscoring its accuracy in determining the physiological significance of coronary stenosis. In a recent randomized trial involving patients with stable angina, a stress CMR strategy resulted in fewer coronary revascularizations compared to invasive FFR, while demonstrating non-inferior cardiac outcomes [26].

Dobutamine stress CMR, which assesses changes in both regional cine function and perfusion, is less frequently used than vasodilating stress CMR perfusion imaging. It is typically reserved for patients who cannot tolerate vasodilating stress infusions but has shown excellent sensitivity and specificity in detecting CAD, regardless of underlying resting wall motion abnormalities. Clinical studies have demonstrated that dobutamine cine CMR provides strong prognostic value in risk assessment. In specialized centers, stress CMR combined with exercise treadmill stress has also shown promising results [27].

4.1.4.2 Myocardial Viability Assessment

The CMR imaging provides a comprehensive assessment of myocardial structure and function, aiding in the evaluation of myocardial viability. The combined use of end-diastolic wall thickness greater than 5.5 mm and cine systolic wall thickening greater than 2 mm offers a reliable prediction of segmental contractile recovery following coronary revascularization, with sensitivity and specificity ranging from 85% to 90% [28].

The LGE imaging plays a crucial role in assessing myocardial scar tissue and effectively depicts the transmural extent of scarring. This assessment reveals a progressive, stepwise decrease in functional recovery, particularly in myocardial regions exhibiting akinesia or dyskinesia, even after successful revascularization. LGE imaging is straightforward to perform and interpret, with a 50% transmurality cutoff being particularly sensitive for detecting the potential for segmental contractile recovery [9].

Low-dose dobutamine cine imaging provides a functional evaluation of mid-myocardial and subepicardial contractile reserve [29]. It can be particularly useful in situations where tissue edema is significant, such as in the early stages following an MI, where infarct transmurality assessment may be challenging.

4.1.4.3 Acute Coronary Syndrome Assessment

CMR imaging offers a comprehensive assessment of myocardial changes resulting from acute coronary syndrome (ACS) in a single session. It evaluates myocardial structure and function through cine cardiac imaging, assesses perfusion, detects infarction using LGE imaging, and measures myocardial edema or other tissue characteristics through T1- or T2-weighted imaging or mapping [9].

LGE imaging is the most sensitive and accurate method for detecting subendocardial infarction and quantifying infarct size, with a spatial resolution of 1.5–2 mm and a high contrast-to-noise ratio [30]. Although CMR is not the first imaging modality following an acute MI, it is invaluable for the assessment of various post-MI concerns, including perfusion status evaluation, assessing the extent of viable myocardium, aneurysm formation, intracavitary thrombus, microvascular obstruction, pericarditis, or ventricular septal defect.

In patients with reperfused MI, CMR techniques such as T1 or T2 mapping, LGE, and T2* mapping can quantify ischemic area-at-risk, microvascular obstruction (no-reflow), and intramyocardial hemorrhage, respectively. Dark-blood LGE imaging enhances the detection of subendocardial infarction by improving the distinction between infarcted tissue and the surrounding blood pool [31].

A small randomized trial has demonstrated that combining CMR with CCTA as a first-line approach reduces the need for invasive angiography without compromising outcomes compared to routine care. CMR is considered the noninvasive gold standard for measuring infarct size and microvascular obstruction, contributing to long-term prognosis and identifying potential benefits of new cardioprotective strategies in clinical trials [32, 33].

For patients with ST-segment elevation myocardial infarction (STEMI) following post-primary percutaneous coronary intervention (PCI), CMR shows moderate to good agreement with invasive FFR assessments of non-culprit coronary lesions [34]. In acute chest pain syndromes, CMR combined with coronary CTA for imaging infarction, myocardial salvage, and coronary stenosis has been shown to enhance the efficiency of invasive coronary angiography [35].

In a cohort of 388 patients with elevated troponins but non-obstructive coronary arteries, CMR identified myocardial inflammation, acute MI, or other cardiomyopathies as the cause of abnormal troponins in about three-fourths of cases. The remaining one-fourth, with no abnormalities detected on CMR, had a favorable prognosis [36]. A recent study involving 229 patients with elevated troponins and non-obstructed coronary arteries demonstrated that a new 3D free-breathing LGE imaging technique achieved an in-plane resolution of 1.3 mm and reduced inconclusive diagnoses by 29% [37].

Non-obstructive CAD is frequently observed in MI patients, affecting 9–20% of females and 4–8% of males [38–40]. While obstructive CAD is associated with a worse prognosis, patients with MI and non-obstructive CAD (MINOCA) have a reinfarction rate of 2–5% [41, 42]. The mechanisms underlying MINOCA are not fully understood, and advanced imaging techniques like intravascular imaging and CMR may help elucidate the etiology. Microvascular coronary disease, known to cause chest pain in the absence of obstructive CAD, could potentially lead to ACS in some MINOCA patients, although this hypothesis requires further investigation [43].

4.1.5 Safety and Practical Considerations

MRI has seen significant advancements in patient safety. Food and Drug Administration-approved MRI-conditional pacemakers and implantable cardioverter defibrillators are devices that enable patients to undergo MRI safely under specific imaging conditions. Established protocols now include device interrogation before and after MRI scanning, allowing many patients with non-MRI-conditional (legacy) devices to undergo CMR in experienced centers. A study of 1509 patients with legacy devices who underwent 2103 MRI studies reported a device reset rate of 0.4%, with only one instance of post-MRI device dysfunction requiring replacement [44].

Additional safety considerations for CMR include various implants. Sternal wires, mechanical heart valves, annuloplasty rings, coronary stents, non-metallic catheters, and orthopedic or dental implants are generally safe for clinical CMR scanning. However, certain implants pose potential hazards, including cochlear implants, neurostimulators, hydrocephalus shunts, metal-containing ocular implants, most breast tissue expanders, and metallic cerebral aneurysm clips.

Claustrophobia, which was once a significant concern, has become less common with the advent of wide-bore MRI scanners. Currently, about 2% of patients experience claustrophobia, which is typically managed effectively with oral sedation administered prior to scanning [45].

4.2 AI Algorithms for Quantifying Myocardial Perfusion

4.2.1 Imaging Methods for Diagnosis of CAD

CAD is characterized by reduced myocardial perfusion, typically due to atherosclerotic plaques in the coronary arteries. While coronary angiography remains the gold-standard diagnostic method for CAD diagnosis, its invasive nature and potential contraindications limit its use in certain patients. To address these limitations, non-invasive quantitative imaging techniques in nuclear cardiology, collectively known as myocardial perfusion imaging (MPI), have been developed to assess myocardial perfusion effectively. The most widely used of these are positron emission tomography (PET) MPI and SPECT MPI, both of which serve as the standard reference methods for the quantitative evaluation of myocardial perfusion under both rest and stress conditions [46]. In addition to SPECT and PET, magnetic resonance (MR) perfusion and CCTA imaging are other techniques for quantitatively assessing myocardial perfusion. However, interpreting SPECT MPI and CCTA results often requires manual classification by expert clinicians, a time-consuming process dependent on the clinician's experience and subject to inter-reader variability.

4.2.2 Incorporation of AI in CAD Diagnosis

Integrating AI algorithms into nuclear cardiology has markedly enhanced the diagnosis and classification of CAD, including myocardial perfusion measurement and calcium scoring. AI models have effectively automatically interpreted SPECT-MPI scintigraphy images [47], CCTA, and MR perfusion. These algorithms, encompassing machine learning (ML) and deep learning (DL) techniques, can be applied to SPECT images to classify perfusion abnormalities and quantify myocardial perfusion. ML algorithms, such as Random Forest (RF), Support Vector Machine (SVM), Logistic Regression, Artificial Neural Networks (ANNs), and eXtreme Gradient Boosting (XGBoost), along with DL models like Generative Adversarial Networks (GANs), Convolutional Neural Networks (CNNs), and Graph CNNs, have demonstrated significant potential in improving the quantification of myocardial perfusion [48]. The deployment of these AI models has instilled confidence in the reliability and accuracy of AI-based CAD diagnosis.

This section reviews the latest advancements in AI algorithms, emphasizing their potential to substantially improve diagnostic accuracy and build trust within the medical community regarding AI-based quantification of myocardial perfusion and CAD diagnosis. It also addresses the challenges associated with AI implementation and explores potential solutions for future improvements.

4.2.2.1 ML Models for Quantifying Myocardial Perfusion

ML algorithms have demonstrated significant potential in detecting perfusion abnormalities in patients with CAD across various studies [49, 50]. Nakajima et al. (2017) [51] developed an ANN model to classify rest/stress tests using SPECT images from 1001 patients. They incorporated additional input data, including PCI history, coronary artery bypass grafting results, risk factors, weight, height, and sex. The ANN model outperformed conventional methods, achieving an area under the curve (AUC) of 0.92 compared to 0.82.

In a 2019 study, Filho et al. utilized an SVM model to classify myocardial ischemia in 82 patients using myocardial perfusion scintigraphy (MPS). The model achieved a concordance rate of 66% compared to the gold-standard technique [52]. In a subsequent study, Filho et al. [53] employed an RF algorithm to classify normal and abnormal CAD cases in 1007 rest/stress SPECT-MPI images. After applying tenfold cross-validation, the RF model achieved a sensitivity of 0.963, a precision of 0.968, an accuracy of 0.93, and an AUC of 0.853.

Arsanjani et al. enhanced an SVM model by integrating left ventricular ejection fraction, ischemic changes, and total perfusion deficit (TPD) and compared it to using TPD alone. The integrated model achieved an accuracy of 86%, surpassing the 81% accuracy of TPD alone [54]. Rahmani et al. [55] constructed an ANN model to predict CAD based on rest and stress MPI images from 93 cases, incorporating clinical data into the analysis. Their model achieved an accuracy of 85.7% in predicting CAD.

CAC scoring, a marker of atherosclerosis and a predictor of adverse cardiac events, is traditionally performed manually by nuclear imaging experts using non-contrast CT. However, recent advances in ML algorithms have enabled automatic CAC scoring, improving clinical workflow and reducing physician workload. Wolterink et al. (2014) [56] developed a supervised RF model to automatically differentiate between non-coronary and coronary calcifications based on cardiac CT exams from 250 patients, with their model showing a strong correlation with expert manual interpretation ($r = 0.94$).

ML networks have also been applied to CCTA images to reduce cardiologists' manual workload and enhance diagnostic accuracy in identifying coronary artery stenosis [57]. For instance, Liang et al. developed an M-Net CNN to automatically measure percentage diameter stenosis and minimal luminal area, achieving a strong correlation ($r = 0.984$) with expert measurements [58]. Similarly, in another study, Han et al. (2018) [59] developed an ML approach to diagnose CAD using CCTA and invasive FFR data from 252 subjects. They demonstrated that incorporating ML-based computed tomography perfusion analysis improved the predictive power for significant ischemia beyond coronary stenosis alone.

4.2.2.2 DL Models for Quantifying Myocardial Perfusion

CNNs have demonstrated high diagnostic accuracy for CAD classification, particularly when applied to SPECT-MPI imaging [60–69]. In a 2022 systematic review and meta-analysis by Alskaf et al. [70], the efficacy of 46 studies utilizing DL models for automatic myocardial perfusion quantification was evaluated. The review reported a pooled diagnostic accuracy of 0.859 for DL models in classifying MPS images. Moreover, CNNs outperformed multi-layer perceptron (MLP) models, achieving a pooled AUC of 0.894 compared to 0.848 for MLPs. While there was no heterogeneity among the studies, a potential publication bias was noted.

In a recent study by Kusumoto et al. (2024) [71], a DL-based diagnostic support system was developed using 5443 SPECT-MPI images. A CNN was trained to classify these images as either healthy or CAD-positive. The CNN's performance was compared with cardiologists using

AI-guided diagnosis and those diagnosing without AI assistance. The CNN achieved an accuracy of 88%, surpassing the AI-assisted cardiologists (80%) and those without AI support (65%). Additionally, the AI-based system reduced the time required for diagnosis by 19 min. The authors concluded that this AI-based system improves diagnostic accuracy and reduces cardiologists' workload.

Similarly, Otaki et al. (2022) [72] developed an explainable DL model to detect obstructive CAD using 3578 stress-mode SPECT-MPI images. The model, evaluated using a tenfold repeated test, achieved a higher AUC (0.9073) than the reader diagnosis (0.71). External validation on a high-CAD-prevalence cohort revealed a per-vessel AUC of 0.78 and a per-patient AUC of 0.80. Chen et al. [73] introduced a 3D-CNN model for cadmium zinc telluride SPECT images from 979 patients, achieving classification specificity, sensitivity, and accuracy of 92.16%, 81.58%, and 87.64%, respectively, using fivefold cross-validation.

In a large-scale study by Liu et al. [74], a DL model named ResNet-34 was utilized to detect abnormal myocardial perfusion in 37,243 patients undergoing stress SPECT-MPI (99mTc-Tetrofosmin or 99mTc-Sestamibi MPI). Additional features such as stress type, radiotracer, length, BMI, and gender were incorporated as secondary inputs. The DL model outperformed the standard quantitative perfusion defect size (DS) method, with an AUC of 0.872 versus 0.838. The authors suggested that DL holds substantial potential for enhancing the diagnostic accuracy of myocardial perfusion abnormalities in stress-only MPI.

Xue et al. (2020) [75] developed a deep neural network (DNN) for segmenting and quantifying myocardial blood flow (MBF) in 1825 MR perfusion series from 1034 patients. The CNN model produced MBF measurements that closely matched those obtained via manual methods, affirming the reliability of AI in CAD diagnosis. Zhang et al. (2023) [76] developed a neural network for 599 patients with hybrid SPECT scans, achieving a precision of 80.17–98.15% and an accuracy of 66.20–94.64% on the training set. The model's validation set AUC and specificity of more than 90%. This model outperformed most interpreters at varying experience levels.

The key consideration in applying AI models for quantifying myocardial perfusion and diagnosing CAD is whether these models can enhance clinicians' performance while reducing analysis time and alleviating cardiologist burnout. In a study by Miller et al. [77], the effectiveness of a CAD-DL model in improving clinicians' interpretation of MPI for obstructive CAD was assessed. The study compared the performance of expert clinicians with and without the CAD-DL algorithm. The results indicated that the AUC increased from 0.747 without CAD-DL to 0.779 with it. Additionally, all clinicians achieved higher accuracy with the CAD-DL model, showing a 0.02–0.05 improvement in AUC. The CAD-DL model also enhanced overall net reclassification by 17.2%.

Garcia et al. [78] took this further by developing an AI-driven structured reporting system that automatically generates reports. The reports were compared to those of expert nuclear cardiologists. The AI-generated reports demonstrated diagnostic performance comparable to that of human experts, reinforcing the potential of DL to improve MPI interpretation.

In addition to conventional ML and DL models, there is growing interest in hybrid multi-input networks, which combine these approaches. Apostolopoulos et al. (2021) [63] explored this by using a hybrid RF-CNN model that incorporated clinical data (e.g., recurrent diseases, predisposing factors, symptoms, gender, and age) to diagnose CAD from stress and rest scintigraphic MPI polar map images. The model, which used the CNN (InceptionV3) algorithm, achieved an AUC of 0.7915, similar to the accuracy of expert interpretation.

Another advancement in AI applications is transfer learning, which improves a model's performance for similar tasks on different datasets. Papandrianos et al. (2021) [79] applied transfer learning to diagnose infarction or ischemia, achieving an AUC of 0.936 and a classification accuracy of 93.47% ± 2.81%. Their robust DL models utilized various pre-trained networks, such as InceptionV3 and DenseNet, alongside data augmentation to expand the dataset.

In another study by Papandrianos et al. [80], the authors evaluated the performance of a CNN model on SPECT-MPI for classifying cases into normal/abnormal. Their model showed excellent results with 90.21% accuracy and 0.937 AUC.

Myocardial perfusion reserve index (MPRI) is an important indicator of ischemia on MRI, which usually requires manual adjustment. Kim et al. (2023) [81] developed a fully automatic U-Net algorithm with ML landmark detection to estimate the MPRI on dynamic contrast-enhanced MRI. Using the proposed model, the MPRI measurement correlated with results from the manual reference (P-value <0.001). Although results showed superior performance of manual MPRI measurement, this method still holds the potential to measure myocardial ischemia quantitatively.

Like the ML models described earlier, DL models have also shown promising results in automatic CAC scoring in cardiovascular disease subjects [82, 83]. In a study by Zeleznik et al. [84], the authors used a U-Net CNN network to quantify CAC scores automatically. Their model showed a strong correlation with manual scoring by the experts (r = 0.92). Moreover, DL models can also be used to quantify stenosis and plaque using CCTA images. In another study by Velzen et al. (2020) [83], the authors developed a DL model for automatic CAC scoring based on CT images. Their DL model showed an intraclass correlation coefficient of 0.79–0.97 for CAC and achieved an AUC of 0.93.

DL models have also been applied to CCTA images for CAD diagnosis. In a study, Lin et al. [85] used a CNN network to quantify atherosclerotic plaque as a tool for CAD diagnosis. Experiments demonstrated that their proposed CNN rapidly quantifies stenosis severity and plaque volume on CCTA. Their model also closely agreed with intravascular ultrasound and expert readers' estimation. Their model also showed good prognostic potential for future MI.

In addition to MPI-SPECT and CCTA, DL algorithms could also be applied to CMR images to facilitate the quantification of myocardial blood flow. Knott et al. [86] applied their AI model to a dataset of 1049 CMRs of suspected or known CAD patients. They observed that their model could effectively quantify the reduced myocardial blood flow and strongly predict adverse cardiovascular events.

4.3 AI-Driven Magnetic Resonance Imaging for Identifying Ischemia and Infarction

4.3.1 Role of CMR in Cardiac Imaging

The European Society of Cardiology 2017 and the Society for Cardiovascular Magnetic Resonance 2020 position paper [87] endorse CMR as a significant cardiac imaging technique for evaluating the prognostic impact of myocardial damage following MI [88]. Within clinical trials, CMR is valuable for evaluating the effectiveness of prospective cardioprotective treatments in decreasing the extent of MI and avoiding negative remodeling of the left ventricle (LV) in reperfused MI [89]. Collaborative mapping of native T1, T2, T2*, and post-contrast T1 might provide a more profound understanding of the pathophysiological processes following MI and their related prognostic importance [90, 91].

LGE is the gold standard imaging used to evaluate myocardial scarring and viability on CMR. This assessment is valuable for informing clinical decision-making about revascularization, risk stratification, and long-term prognosis in treating patients with ischemic heart disease (IHD) [92, 93]. CMR can accurately identify subendocardial MI as little as 1 gram in size. It identifies minor and subendocardial infarctions that may go undetected by other imaging modalities [94–96]. Empirical research has demonstrated that the magnitude of infarct size and transmurality on LGE-CMR is indicative of functional enhancement following revascularization [97–99]. However, LGE necessitates the use of intravenous GBCA, which prolongs the scanning duration and is not recommended for some populations. There is a growing movement towards adopting less invasive, contrast-free methods, which can decrease scan and preparation durations, save expenses, and enhance the accessibility of CMR [100].

Furthermore, the process of manually contouring and analyzing can be time-consuming due to the variability between and within observers. This, in turn, might result in a decrease in the accuracy and precision of the analysis [101]. However, the time-consuming nature of CMR interpretation, the significant time and effort required to acquire the necessary skills, and the consequent lack of clinicians with the necessary training have all inhibited the broad clinical deployment of CMR. It may be quite challenging to diagnose cardiovascular diseases (CVDs) using CMR in a timely and accurate manner due to the shortage of specialists with the necessary training. As a result, there is a lot of clinical potential for using automated CMR interpretation for quick CVD screening and diagnosis [102, 103].

Automated imaging analysis methods utilizing AI, particularly DL approaches, can facilitate the creation of efficient, robust, accurate, and clinician-friendly tools. These tools aim to enhance both clinician productivity and overall quality of patient care [104].

4.3.2 AI Applications in CMR

4.3.2.1 Diagnosis of MI

The diagnosis of MI using ML is predominantly applied in CMR [105]. The primary imaging method in CMR is cine sequence, which generates sequential pictures often employed to evaluate the contractile function of the heart. LGE sequence is a widely recognized method for measuring the degree of tissue anomalies in or around the heart muscle. It can be employed to identify and confirm MI [106]. Larroza et al. [107] studied 50 patients with chronic MI using LGE and cine CMR to detect the infarcted nonviable, viable, and distant segments with an AUC of 0.849.

Baessler et al. [108] applied a radiomic technique to detect subacute and chronic MI on non-contrast-enhanced cine CMR, achieving an AUC of 0.93 and 0.92, respectively.

Zhang et al. [105] employed a DL approach to identify chronic MI in 212 individuals using non-enhanced cine CMR. The achieved AUC was 0.94. Numerous studies have demonstrated that a non-enhanced cine CMR may accurately detect MI with comparable effectiveness to LGE CMR. Thus, AI has the capacity to decrease the dosage of gadolinium contrast injection [109].

4.3.2.2 CMR Images Resolution Enhancement

Cardiac MRI images are dynamic 3D pictures with high-resolution in-plane information. Clinical CMR uses high-resolution 2D stacks of images to create anisotropic 3D heart volumes owing to patient breath-hold duration limits. Thus, these 3D volumes have low through-plane resolution [110], which makes image viewing, analysis, and diagnosis challenging [111]. Interpolation methods, while commonly used, introduce blurring and information loss and thus cannot fully resolve this issue. To overcome this problem, researchers have suggested super-resolution technologies that computationally enhance image resolution [110].

In recent years, there has been an increase in the use of deep neural network-based image super-resolution techniques to improve the resolution of MRI images [112]. Successful use of DL-based super-resolution approaches to cine CMR images has been observed [113]. For instance, Steeden et al. [114] demonstrated the capability of a 3D residual U-Net architecture to achieve super-resolution by utilizing synthetic whole-heart images captured during balanced steady-state free precession sequences.

However, acquiring high-resolution isotropic images from real-world data for training supervised models remains challenging. To overcome this, Bustin et al. [115] introduced an innovative method for reconstructing 3D LGE CMR images by utilizing a 3D self-similarity framework. Additionally, Upendra et al. offer a self-supervised DL approach for super-resolution LGE CMR images. No external training data is needed since this approach improves through-plane resolution using high-resolution in-plane data. The suggested approach is tested on the 2018 atrial segmentation challenge dataset [110, 116].

4.3.2.3 Image Segmentation

Segmentation, which involves manually contouring the borders of the cardiac chambers and myocardium, is a time-consuming procedure. Moreover, there might still exist inconsistencies in the results of the analysis among professional observers. ML techniques can be employed to automate image segmentation and enhance productivity, accuracy, and consistency [117]. This may be accomplished by either pixel-wise categorization or regression-based methods. Fully automated myocardial segmentation has great potential for more time-efficient postprocessing with automated delivery of prognostically relevant CMR parameters, which may allow broad adoption of risk stratification without impeding diagnostic workflow in clinical practice [118].

Schuster et al. [118] demonstrated that a fully automated volumetric analysis of MI using CMR is feasible and can predict major adverse cardiac events with accuracy comparable to traditional volumetric analysis.

The Multimodal RU-Net model by Hong et al. [119] improves the segmentation of edema and scar areas in CMR images by enhancing feature extraction and focusing attention on key regions. It uses a multimodal feature extraction module and attention mechanisms to improve accuracy. Tested on the MyoPS2020 dataset, it achieved stable, competitive performance, making it valuable for automatic myocardial pathology segmentation.

4.3.2.4 Pattern Recognition in LGE Imaging

Myocardial LGE pattern can distinguish ischemic from non-ischemic heart disease with high accuracy, and it can assist in diagnosing cardiomyopathies. In distinct cardiomyopathies, LGE patterns, intramyocardial distribution, and extent have varying prognostic roles [120].

Fahmy et al. [121] have introduced a new method for LGE that utilizes deep CNNs to automatically measure LV mass and scar volume on LGE images in patients with hypertrophic cardiomyopathy. Current methods for manually delineating scar volume, commonly used in standard clinical practice, are subjective, time-consuming, and labor-intensive. Furthermore, even when employing existing thresholding methods for quantifying LGE, accuracy and repeatability are still influenced by differences between data centers, changes in gadolinium kinetics, and dispersed patterns of LGE distribution [122].

4.3.2.5 Infarct Size and Transmurality

Zhang et al. [105] have shown the application of a DL framework on non-contrast cine CMR to validate, identify, and define the transmurality and size of chronic MI. These findings have significant benefits, especially for patients with renal dysfunction who may be unable to get gadolinium contrast yet may need to evaluate myocardial viability using CMR [123].

Chen et al. [124] proposed a CNN-based automated MI segmentation technique for analyzing CMR LGE sequences. Their methodology showed promising segmentation outcomes, outperforming the variability observed in both intra-observer and inter-observer manual segmentations, as well as automatic segmentation using the Gaussian Mixture Model. Kotu et al. [125] utilized pixel intensity and texture-based features to delineate distinct cardiac segments, including the core and border regions affected by MI scarring. In another study, Kotu et al. [126] successfully segmented scarred and non-scarred myocardium in MI patients using various feature combinations within a Bayes classifier. Their results demonstrated equivalence to manual segmentation in all cross-validation scenarios.

Engan et al. [127] developed an experimental framework to explore data by calculating a large number of features to characterize regions of interest in CMR images. Their study found that incorporating texture analysis enhances the ability to differentiate between scarred and non-scarred myocardium, enabling the identification of patients at high and low risk for severe ventricular arrhythmias following MI.

Larroza et al. [128] used ML methods and texture features from CMR imaging scans to distinguish between acute and chronic MI. They concluded that texture analysis could differentiate between acute and chronic MI on both LGE and standard cine sequences, even when infarction is not visually apparent. In another study, Larroza et al. [107] applied texture analysis to distinguish between infarcted nonviable, viable, and distant myocardial sections in MI.

Baessler et al. [108] conducted a proof-of-concept study using stepwise dimension reduction and texture feature selection to diagnose MI from non-enhanced cine images, with LGE serving as the reference standard. Their findings provided empirical evidence supporting the viability of texture analysis for accurately diagnosing subacute and chronic ischemic scars, including small and large infarcts, on non-enhanced cine CMR images.

AI-based virtual native enhancement (VNE) in CMR can accurately detect and display myocardial scars in MI patients. VNE enhances original T1 maps and cine images with DL to create LGE-like images. The initial validation of VNE in hypertrophic cardiomyopathy patients showed high visuospatial agreement with traditional LGE and improved image quality. VNE enables rapid MRI without the need for contrast agents, making it applicable for other conditions in clinical practice, such as myocardial scarring and viability in patients with prior MI, which constitute a significant portion of routine CMR referrals [129, 130]. VNE had better image quality than LGE and was associated substantially with it in assessing scar size and transmurality on 4271 data sets from 912 individuals. The first proof-of-principle comparison of VNE with histopathology in two porcine MI models demonstrated good visuospatial agreement. This research shows that the self-supervised CNN-based super-resolution framework can increase LGE CMR through-plane resolution [100].

4.4 Prognostic Models: Predicting CAD Outcomes with AI

4.4.1 Prognostic Models for CAD from Past to Present

CAD is associated with a significant increase in healthcare costs due to its high morbidity and mortality [131]. It accompanies an increased incidence of major adverse cardiac events (MACE), including MI, stroke, heart failure, and cardiac death. The aim of goal-directed medical interventions that can change the natural trajectory of CAD to a less morbid course is supported by current societal guidelines, which highlight the significance of early detection and risk stratification in the appropriate age and risk groups [132].

Historically, patient-level data that are easily retrieved and helpful to use in the clinical context have been the foundation of traditional population-derived primary and secondary prevention cardiovascular risk assessment methods (e.g., Framingham risk score, ASCVD, TIMI score, GRACE score, etc.). These tools, although significant, are intrinsically constrained by design because they rely on regression models that make numerous mathematical assumptions that are frequently not true in practice, such as homogeneity of effects and collinearity between variables. Such regression-based techniques are less generalizable across diverse groups due to the multifactorial etiology and complicated nature of CAD [131].

AI models utilizing ML and DL can achieve a high level of precision in identifying high-risk patients and forecasting MACE. The purpose of this chapter is to explore how AI models can be used for predicting outcomes in CAD patients, emphasizing the types of models, data sources, and real-world applications.

4.4.2 AI-Based Risk Stratification Models for MACE

Combining clinical, genetic, and imaging data, AI models of MACE risk estimation offer more comprehensive risk assessment information compared to traditional scores. For example, merging genetic and clinical risk factors has been shown to improve the prediction of coronary heart disease [133]. In another study by Amer et al., the AtheroEdge-MCDLAI (AE3.0DL) platform was introduced, leveraging multiclass DL techniques. The study utilized data from 500 patients who underwent both carotid ultrasound and coronary angiography, with stenosis measurements serving as the gold standard. The analysis involved 39 covariates categorized into office-based (e.g., age, BMI, blood pressure), laboratory-based (e.g., hyperlipidemia, kidney function), and carotid ultrasound metrics (e.g., plaque height, area). AE3.0DL employed Recurrent Neural Networks (RNN) and Long Short-Term Memory (LSTM) models, addressing class imbalance using the Synthetic Minority Over-sampling Technique. Performance was evaluated through tenfold cross-validation, yielding accuracy rates of 95% with an AUC of 0.98 for RNN and 95.34% with an AUC of 0.99 for LSTM. These results demonstrate a notable improvement of 32.93% over conventional methods and 9.94% over other ML models, with the platform delivering results in less than 1 s. This advancement underscores the efficacy of DL algorithms in enhancing CAD risk prediction and CVD risk stratification [134].

4.4.3 AI in Cardiovascular Imaging for Predicting MACE

AI models that incorporate advanced imaging data can identify high-risk plaque characteristics and myocardial perfusion abnormalities, enhancing the prediction of future MACE. AI's application in cardiovascular imaging has significantly improved the prognostic accuracy for MACE. Diller et al. investigated the role of AI in analyzing CMR data to predict mortality and MACE in patients with Tetralogy of Fallot. The study showed that AI-generated LV volumetric parameters were highly consistent with manually obtained measurements, underscoring the reliability of AI in delivering accurate prognostic insights [135]. In another study, Slomka et al. established the REFINE SPECT registry, a large, multi-center database designed to promote the advancement of AI in non-invasive imaging. The registry gathers nuclear imaging and clinical data, ensuring pseudo-anonymization and standardized analysis, with follow-up data on MACE. This initiative facilitates the development and validation of AI-based tools for automated diagnosis and risk stratification [136]. AI has also been utilized in the analysis of echocardiography, coronary angiography, and PET imaging to detect early indicators of MACE, such as LV hypertrophy or myocardial fibrosis. These applications underscore the potential of AI to enhance the precision, efficiency, and reproducibility of cardiovascular imaging.

The incorporation of AI, particularly ML and DL, into the diagnosis and management of CAD and MACE holds substantial promise for advancing cardiovascular care. By integrating clinical, genetic, and imaging data, AI-driven models are poised to offer more precise and personalized risk assessments, thereby improving patient outcomes. As AI technology continues to evolve, its role in cardiovascular medicine will likely expand, offering unprecedented opportunities for enhancing the diagnosis and management of CAD and MACE.

4.4.4 AI-Assisted Plaque Assessment for CAD Prognosis

Defining the plaque morphology and estimating the severity of stenosis is possible with the application of AI in computed tomography angiography (CTA) [137].

In a 2024 systematic review and meta-analysis, Pingping et al. assessed the diagnostic accuracy of AI-assisted CCTA for identifying atherosclerotic plaques by examining 11 studies. The combined area under the receiver operating characteristic curve (AUROC) for plaque evaluation was 0.96 (95% CI 0.94–0.97). For detecting stenosis of 50% or more, the AUROC was 0.95 (95% CI 0.93–0.96) from five studies, and for stenosis of 70% or more, it was 0.96 (95% CI 0.94–0.97) from six studies. Additionally, for calcium detection, the AUROC was 0.92 (95% CI 0.90–0.94) from six studies. The study concludes that AI-assisted CTA provides high diagnostic accuracy in detecting stenosis and characterizing plaque, with the best performance for detecting stenosis of 70% or more [138].

In a 2020 study, an end-to-end AI-based tool was evaluated for automated plaque volume analysis, characterization, and high-risk plaque detection in 94 patients using CCTA. The AI tool processed scans in an average of 10.6 ± 2.3 min and identified high-risk plaques in 21% of patients and 9% of vessels, slightly exceeding the expert readers' (Level III) identification rates of 18% and 7%, respectively. The AI analysis strongly correlated with CAD-RADS scores ($r^2 = 0.94$) and detected significant plaque in 50% of cases missed by the experts. Overall, the AI system provided rapid and accurate plaque assessments, closely aligning with expert evaluations [139]. Similarly, Masuda et al. developed an ML model that analyzed histograms of 78 coronary plaques using CCTA, validated against integrated backscatter intravascular ultrasound. The model demonstrated superior diagnostic accuracy compared to traditional CCTA parameters, with an AUC of 0.92 versus 0.83 ($p = 0.001$) [140].

ML techniques, including texture analysis on cardiac CT, are being used for prognosis and MI diagnosis. Preliminary results from the SMARTool Project introduced a novel approach for diagnosing, prognosticating, and treating CAD, combining computational biomechanics and ML-based risk classification. The ML analysis distinguished between low and medium-to-high-risk patients using retrospective and prospective data. CAD diagnosis was supported by 3D coronary artery reconstructions and noninvasive smartFFR estimation [141]. Furthermore, AI is emerging as a transformative tool for predicting all-cause mortality in CAD. In a recent study by Motwani et al., the Logit-Boost classification algorithm was used to predict 5-year mortality in CAD patients. Prior to building the ML model, feature selection was performed using information gain ranking, with only variables contributing to outcome prediction (information gain >0) being included. Of the 25 clinical and 44 CCTA parameters collected, 19 clinical and 35 CCTA variables were chosen for model development. The model, trained and validated through tenfold cross-validation, achieved an AUC of 0.79, outperforming both the Framingham risk score (AUC 0.61) and CCTA severity scores (AUC 0.62–0.64) [142]. This predictive model enabled physicians to make more informed decisions, supporting patient-specific therapy. Overall, predictive modeling for individualized care shows significant potential to enhance data-driven, patient-centered healthcare, improving care standards in the future [143].

AI is also applied for the evaluation of coronary artery stenosis. Zreik et al. developed a 3D CNN for characterizing plaque and assessing stenosis severity. They created two models: the first model evaluated the algorithm's ability to distinguish between patients with and without obstructive CAD, achieving accuracies of 0.94, 0.93, and 0.85 per segment, vessel, and patient, respectively. The second model classified the presence of no stenosis, non-significant stenosis, and significant stenosis, with accuracies of 0.80, 0.76, and 0.75 per segment, vessel, and patient, respectively [144]. Yoneyama et al. explored the potential for evaluating coronary stenosis grading and its impact on ischemia using a cohort of patients who underwent both CCTA and myocardial perfusion SPECT [17]. The study focused on employing an ANN model that combined CCTA with myocardial perfusion SPECT imaging. The algorithm demonstrated a specificity of 31%, a sensitivity of 78%, and an accuracy of 67% in identifying coronary artery stenosis greater than 70% [145]. Van Hamersvelt et al. created an AI algorithm designed to assess the presence of significant CAD by integrating myocardial data and comparing the results with invasive FFR measurements. Their study revealed that this combined approach achieved an AUC of 0.76 for identifying hemodynamically significant CAD [146].

4.5 Integration of AI in the Clinical Management of CAD

Effective management of CAD requires advanced, data-driven approaches. The integration of AI into clinical workflows has introduced transformative possibilities, significantly enhancing the precision and efficiency of decision-making in CAD management.

4.5.1 Early Detection and Risk Assessment

AI systems excel in analyzing large, complex datasets, including patient medical histories, laboratory results, imaging findings, risk factors, and genetic predispositions to CAD. This capability enables early detection and risk assessment, which are critical for implementing effective medical therapies to slow disease progression. For example, CAC—a robust marker of atherosclerosis and a predictor of obstructive CAD—can now be quantified using AI-driven workflows. These automated workflows leverage DL techniques to streamline CAC scoring, reducing the time and effort required compared to traditional manual processes.

4.5.2 Personalized Prognosis and Treatment

AI enhances the integration of cardiovascular magnetic resonance (CMR) imaging with clinical data to predict CAD prognosis and guide personalized treatment strategies. By combining patient histories, imaging findings, and genetic predispositions, AI models can assess the risk of adverse cardiac events and optimize therapeutic approaches. Additionally, AI can monitor CAD progression by comparing new CMR images with prior ones, detecting subtle changes in blood flow, tissue composition, and myocardial strain [147].

4.5.3 Streamlining Imaging Workflows

AI-driven innovations have revolutionized imaging workflows by automating processes that were previously time-intensive. For instance, CNNs enable automatic segmentation of the myocardium during stress perfusion CMR, producing detailed perfusion maps and metrics such as myocardial blood flow and myocardial perfusion reserve. These automated approaches generate results comparable to traditional manual methods while significantly improving efficiency [148].

4.6 Current Challenges and Future Directions

Developing effective ML and DL models hinges on training with large datasets. However, many studies in this area are based on small datasets, which can lead to underfitting and limit the models' generalizability. One major issue is the limited availability of high-quality, annotated datasets, which are crucial for training and validating AI models. Additionally, variability in imaging protocols across institutions leads to inconsistent data, making it difficult for AI algorithms to generalize effectively. To address these challenges, multicenter studies are needed to evaluate the efficacy of DL models on larger, more diverse datasets. Transfer learning, which involves applying a trained model to a different dataset, is another promising approach to improve model performance. Additionally, data augmentation techniques can help mitigate the challenges associated with small datasets by artificially increasing the amount of training data.

One other significant challenge in applying AI models for CAD classification is the "black box" nature of these models, meaning their internal decision-making processes are often opaque due to complex computational functions. Clinicians need transparency and trust in AI-driven decisions for prognosis and treatment planning. Few studies have employed explainable AI (XAI) methods, which are crucial for identifying the regions contributing to predictions, minimizing bias, and enhancing model transparency and interpretability. Future research should prioritize developing and applying XAI techniques to make AI-driven CAD diagnosis more trustworthy and understandable [72].

References

1. Murray CJ, Lopez AD. Alternative projections of mortality and disability by cause 1990–2020: global burden of disease study. Lancet. 1997;349(9064):1498–504.
2. Roger VL, et al. Heart disease and stroke statistics—2011 update: a report from the American Heart Association. Circulation. 2011;123(4):e18–e209.
3. World Health Organization. World health statistics 2008. World Health Organization; 2008.
4. Rezaei M, et al. Role of artificial intelligence in the diagnosis and treatment of diseases. Kindle. 2023;3(1):1–160.
5. Bonow RO, et al. Braunwald's heart disease e-book: A textbook of cardiovascular medicine. Elsevier Health Sciences; 2011.
6. Levitt MH. Spin dynamics: basics of nuclear magnetic resonance. Wiley; 2008.
7. Bottomley PA, et al. A review of normal tissue hydrogen NMR relaxation times and relaxation mechanisms from 1–100 MHz: dependence on tissue type, NMR frequency, temperature, species, excision, and age. Med Phys. 1984;11(4):425–48.
8. Bansal R, et al. The effects of changing water content, relaxation times, and tissue contrast on tissue segmentation and measures of cortical anatomy in MR images. Magn Reson Imaging. 2013;31(10):1709–30.
9. Uhlig J, et al. Gadolinium-based contrast agents for cardiac MRI: use of linear and macrocyclic agents with associated safety profile from 154 779 European patients. Radiol Cardiothorac Imaging. 2020;2(5):e200102.
10. Ferrari V. The EACVI textbook of cardiovascular magnetic resonance. Oxford University Press; 2018.
11. Pasquini L, et al. Gadolinium-based contrast agent-related toxicities. CNS Drugs. 2018;32:229–40.
12. Holland AE, Goldfarb JW, Edelman RR. Diaphragmatic and cardiac motion during suspended breathing: preliminary experience and implications for breath-hold MR imaging. Radiology. 1998;209(2):483–9.
13. Myerson SG, Francis J, Neubauer S. Cardiovascular magnetic resonance. Oxford University Press; 2013.
14. Götte MJ, et al. Myocardial strain and torsion quantified by cardiovascular magnetic resonance tissue tagging: studies in normal and impaired left ventricular function. J Am Coll Cardiol. 2006;48(10):2002–11.
15. Bhuva AN, et al. T1 mapping: non-invasive evaluation of myocardial tissue composition by cardiovascular magnetic resonance. Expert Rev Cardiovasc Ther. 2014;12(12):1455–64.
16. Fratz S, et al. Guidelines and protocols for cardiovascular magnetic resonance in children and adults with congenital heart disease: SCMR expert consensus group on congenital heart disease. J Cardiovasc Magn Reson. 2013;15:1–26.
17. Friedrich MG, Kim HW, Kim RJ. T2-weighted imaging to assess post-infarct myocardium at risk. JACC Cardiovasc Imaging. 2011;4(9):1014–21.
18. Chen D. Improved quantification of myocardial perfusion imaging using MRI. Northwestern University; 2015.
19. Domanski MJ, et al. Time course of LDL cholesterol exposure and cardiovascular disease event risk. J Am Coll Cardiol. 2020;76(13):1507–16.
20. Lakatta EG. So! what's aging? Is cardiovascular aging a disease? J Mol Cell Cardiol. 2015;83:1–13.
21. Coelho-Filho OR, et al. Stress myocardial perfusion imaging by CMR provides strong prognostic value to cardiac events regardless of patient's sex. JACC Cardiovasc Imaging. 2011;4(8):850–61.
22. Mozaffarian D, et al. Heart disease and stroke statistics—2016 update: a report from the American Heart Association. Circulation. 2016;133(4):e38–e360.
23. Forman DE, et al. Multimorbidity in older adults with cardiovascular disease. J Am Coll Cardiol. 2018;71(19):2149–61.
24. Forman DE, et al. Prioritizing functional capacity as a principal end point for therapies oriented to older adults with cardiovascular disease: a scientific statement for healthcare professionals from the American Heart Association. Circulation. 2017;135(16):e894–918.
25. Paneni F, et al. The aging cardiovascular system: understanding it at the cellular and clinical levels. J Am Coll Cardiol. 2017;69(15):1952–67.
26. Ferrucci L, Fabbri E. Inflammageing: chronic inflammation in ageing, cardiovascular disease, and frailty. Nat Rev Cardiol. 2018;15(9):505–22.
27. Aronow WS, et al. ACCF/AHA 2011 expert consensus document on hypertension in the elderly: a report of the American College of Cardiology Foundation task force on clinical expert consensus documents. Circulation. 2011;123(21):2434–506.
28. Eitel I, et al. Comprehensive prognosis assessment by CMR imaging after ST-segment elevation myocardial infarction. J Am Coll Cardiol. 2014;64(12):1217–26.
29. Valente FX, et al. Predictive value of cardiac magnetic resonance feature tracking after acute myocardial infarction: a comparison with dobutamine stress echocardiography. J Clin Med. 2021;10(22):5261.

30. Toupin S, et al. Whole-heart high-resolution late gadolinium enhancement: techniques and clinical applications. J Magn Reson Imaging. 2022;55(4):967–87.
31. Fleg JL, Strait J. Age-associated changes in cardiovascular structure and function: a fertile milieu for future disease. Heart Fail Rev. 2012;17:545–54.
32. Addison O, et al. Intermuscular fat: a review of the consequences and causes. Int J Endocrinol. 2014;2014(1):309570.
33. Kitzman DW, et al. Skeletal muscle abnormalities and exercise intolerance in older patients with heart failure and preserved ejection fraction. Am J Phys Heart Circ Phys. 2014;306(9):H1364–70.
34. Arnett DK, et al. AHA/ACC/HHS strategies to enhance application of clinical practice guidelines in patients with cardiovascular disease and comorbid conditions: from the American Heart Association, American College of Cardiology, and US Department of Health and Human Services. Circulation. 2014;130(18):1662–7.
35. Afilalo J, et al. Frailty assessment in the cardiovascular care of older adults. J Am Coll Cardiol. 2014;63(8):747–62.
36. Boccardi V, Mecocci P. The importance of cellular senescence in frailty and cardiovascular diseases. In: Frailty and cardiovascular diseases: research into an elderly population. Cham: Springer; 2020. p. 79–86.
37. Forman DE, Alexander KP. Frailty: a vital sign for older adults with cardiovascular disease. Can J Cardiol. 2016;32(9):1082–7.
38. Berger JS, et al. Sex differences in mortality following acute coronary syndromes. JAMA. 2009;302(8):874–82.
39. Halkin A, et al. Outcomes of patients consented but not randomized in a trial of primary percutaneous coronary intervention in acute myocardial infarction (the CADILLAC registry). Am J Cardiol. 2005;96(12):1649–55.
40. Js H. Sex, clinical presentation, and outcomes in patients with acute coronary syndromes. N Engl J Med. 1999;341:226–32.
41. Dey S, et al. Sex-related differences in the presentation, treatment and outcomes among patients with acute coronary syndromes: the global registry of acute coronary events. Heart. 2009;95(1):20–6.
42. Diver DJ, et al. Clinical and arteriographic characterization of patients with unstable angina without critical coronary arterial narrowing (from the TIMI-IIIA trial). Am J Cardiol. 1994;74(6):531–7.
43. Reynolds HR, et al. Mechanisms of myocardial infarction in women without angiographically obstructive coronary artery disease. Circulation. 2011;124(13):1414–25.
44. Symons R, Zimmerman SL, Bluemke DA. CMR and CT of the patient with cardiac devices: safety, efficacy, and optimization strategies. JACC Cardiovasc Imaging. 2019;12(5):890–903.
45. Nguyen K-L, et al. Safety and tolerability of regadenoson CMR. Eur Heart J Cardiovasc Imaging. 2014;15(7):753–60.
46. El-Tallawi KC, et al. Myocardial perfusion imaging using positron emission tomography. Methodist Debakey Cardiovasc J. 2020;16(2):114–21.
47. van der Bijl P, Stassen J, Bax JJ. Application of a deep learning algorithm to calcium scoring in myocardial perfusion imaging. J Nucl Cardiol. 2023;30(1):321–3.
48. Papandrianos NI, et al. AI-based classification algorithms in SPECT myocardial perfusion imaging for cardiovascular diagnosis: a review. Nucl Med Commun. 2023;44(1):1–11.
49. Baskaran L, et al. Machine learning insight into the role of imaging and clinical variables for the prediction of obstructive coronary artery disease and revascularization: an exploratory analysis of the CONSERVE study. PLoS One. 2020;15(6):e0233791.
50. Miller RJH, et al. Machine learning to predict abnormal myocardial perfusion from pre-test features. J Nucl Cardiol. 2022;29(5):2393–403.
51. Nakajima K, et al. Diagnostic accuracy of an artificial neural network compared with statistical quantitation of myocardial perfusion images: a Japanese multicenter study. Eur J Nucl Med Mol Imaging. 2017;44(13):2280–9.
52. Souza-Filho EMD, et al. Artificial intelligence tools for the evaluation of myocardial perfusion imaging. J Nucl Med. 2019;60(Suppl 1):1442.
53. de Souza Filho EM, et al. Machine learning algorithms to distinguish myocardial perfusion SPECT polar maps. Front Cardiovasc Med. 2021;8:741667.
54. Arsanjani R, et al. Improved accuracy of myocardial perfusion SPECT for the detection of coronary artery disease using a support vector machine algorithm. J Nucl Med. 2013;54(4):549–55.
55. Rahmani R, et al. Precisión diagnóstica mejorada para la imagen de perfusión miocárdica usando redes neuronales artificiales en diferentes variables de entrada incluyendo datos clínicos y de cuantificación. Rev Esp Med Nucl Imagen Mol. 2019;38(5):275–9.
56. Wolterink J, et al. An automatic machine learning system for coronary calcium scoring in clinical non-contrast enhanced, ECG-triggered cardiac CT. Med Imaging. 2014;9035
57. Xiong G, et al. Myocardial perfusion analysis in cardiac computed tomography angiographic images at rest. Med Image Anal. 2015;24(1):77–89.
58. Choi AD, et al. CT evaluation by artificial intelligence for atherosclerosis, stenosis and vascular morphology (CLARIFY): a multi-center, international study. J Cardiovasc Comput Tomogr. 2021;15(6):470–6.
59. Han D, et al. Incremental role of resting myocardial computed tomography perfusion for predicting physiologically significant coronary artery disease: a machine learning approach. J Nucl Cardiol. 2018;25(1):223–33.

60. Spier N, et al. Classification of polar maps from cardiac perfusion imaging with graph-convolutional neural networks. Sci Rep. 2019;9(1):7569.
61. Kaplan Berkaya S, Ak Sivrikoz I, Gunal S. Classification models for SPECT myocardial perfusion imaging. Comput Biol Med. 2020;123:103893.
62. Betancur J, et al. Deep learning for prediction of obstructive disease from fast myocardial perfusion SPECT: a multicenter study. JACC Cardiovasc Imaging. 2018;11(11):1654–63.
63. Apostolopoulos ID, et al. Multi-input deep learning approach for cardiovascular disease diagnosis using myocardial perfusion imaging and clinical data. Phys Med. 2021;84:168–77.
64. Zahiri N, et al. Deep learning analysis of polar maps from SPECT myocardial perfusion imaging for prediction of coronary artery disease. Res Square; 2021.
65. Apostolopoulos ID, et al. Deep learning-enhanced nuclear medicine SPECT imaging applied to cardiac studies. EJNMMI Phys. 2023;10(1):6.
66. Trung NT, et al. A deeplearning method for diagnosing coronary artery disease using SPECT images of heart. J Sci Technol. 2020;144:022–7.
67. Arvidsson I, et al. Prediction of obstructive coronary artery disease from myocardial perfusion scintigraphy using deep. Neural Netw. 2021:4442–9.
68. Papandrianos NI, et al. Deep learning-based automated diagnosis for coronary artery disease using SPECT-MPI images. J Clin Med. 2022;11(13)
69. Papandrianos NI, et al. Deep learning exploration for SPECT MPI polar map images classification in coronary artery disease. Ann Nucl Med. 2022;36(9):823–33.
70. Alskaf E, et al. Deep learning applications in myocardial perfusion imaging, a systematic review and meta-analysis. Informat Med Unlocked. 2022;32:101055.
71. Kusumoto D, et al. A deep learning-based automated diagnosis system for SPECT myocardial perfusion imaging. Sci Rep. 2024;14(1):13583.
72. Otaki Y, et al. Clinical deployment of explainable artificial intelligence of SPECT for diagnosis of coronary artery disease. JACC Cardiovasc Imaging. 2022;15(6):1091–102.
73. Chen J-J, et al. Convolutional neural network in the evaluation of myocardial ischemia from CZT SPECT myocardial perfusion imaging: comparison to automated quantification. Appl Sci. 2021;11(2):514.
74. Liu H, et al. Diagnostic accuracy of stress-only myocardial perfusion SPECT improved by deep learning. Eur J Nucl Med Mol Imaging. 2021;48(9):2793–800.
75. Xue H, et al. Automated inline analysis of myocardial perfusion MRI with deep learning. Radiol Artif Intell. 2020;2(6):e200009.
76. Shen LS, et al. A diagnostic method for cardiomyopathy based on multimodal data. Biomed Eng Biomed Tech. 2023;68(4):411–20.
77. Miller RJH, et al. Explainable deep learning improves physician interpretation of myocardial perfusion imaging. J Nucl Med. 2022;63(11):1768–74.
78. Garcia EV, et al. Diagnostic performance of an artificial intelligence-driven cardiac-structured reporting system for myocardial perfusion SPECT imaging. J Nucl Cardiol. 2020;27(5):1652–64.
79. Apostolopoulos ID, et al. Automatic characterization of myocardial perfusion imaging polar maps employing deep learning and data augmentation. Hell J Nucl Med. 2020;23(2):125–32.
80. Papandrianos N, Feleki A, Papageorgiou E. Exploring classification of SPECT MPI images applying convolutional neural networks. In: Proceedings of the 25th Pan-Hellenic Conference on Informatics. Volos, Greece: Association for Computing Machinery; 2022. p. 483–9.
81. Kim Y-C, Kim K, Choe YH. Automatic calculation of myocardial perfusion reserve using deep learning with uncertainty quantification. Quant Imaging Med Surg. 2023;13(12):7936–49.
82. de Vos BD, et al. Direct automatic coronary calcium scoring in cardiac and chest CT. IEEE Trans Med Imaging. 2019;38(9):2127–38.
83. van Velzen SGM, et al. Deep learning for automatic calcium scoring in CT: validation using multiple cardiac CT and chest CT protocols. Radiology. 2020;295(1):66–79.
84. Zeleznik R, et al. Deep convolutional neural networks to predict cardiovascular risk from computed tomography. Nat Commun. 2021;12(1):715.
85. Lin A, et al. Deep learning-enabled coronary CT angiography for plaque and stenosis quantification and cardiac risk prediction: an international multicentre study. Lancet Digit Health. 2022;4(4):e256–65.
86. Knott KD, et al. The prognostic significance of quantitative myocardial perfusion: an artificial intelligence-based approach using perfusion mapping. Circulation. 2020;141(16):1282–91.
87. Leiner T, et al. SCMR position paper (2020) on clinical indications for cardiovascular magnetic resonance. J Cardiovasc Magn Reson. 2020;22(1):76.
88. Ibanez B, et al. 2017 ESC guidelines for the management of acute myocardial infarction in patients presenting with ST-segment elevation: the task force for the management of acute myocardial infarction in patients presenting with ST-segment elevation of the European Society of Cardiology (ESC). Eur Heart J. 2018;39(2):119–77.
89. Bulluck H, et al. Myocardial infarct size by CMR in clinical cardioprotection studies: insights from randomized controlled trials. JACC Cardiovasc Imaging. 2017;10(3):230–40.
90. Messroghli DR, et al. Clinical recommendations for cardiovascular magnetic resonance mapping of T1, T2, T2* and extracellular volume: a consensus statement by the Society for Cardiovascular Magnetic Resonance (SCMR) endorsed by the European Association for Cardiovascular Imaging (EACVI). J Cardiovasc Magn Reson. 2016;19(1):75.

91. Bulluck H, et al. Cardiovascular magnetic resonance in acute st-segment–elevation myocardial infarction: recent advances, controversies, and future directions. Circulation. 2018;137(18):1949–64.
92. Roes SD, et al. Comparison of myocardial infarct size assessed with contrast-enhanced magnetic resonance imaging and left ventricular function and volumes to predict mortality in patients with healed myocardial infarction. Am J Cardiol. 2007;100(6):930–6.
93. Kelle S, et al. Prognostic value of myocardial infarct size and contractile reserve using magnetic resonance imaging. J Am Coll Cardiol. 2009;54(19):1770–7.
94. Kim HW, Farzaneh-Far A, Kim RJ. Cardiovascular magnetic resonance in patients with myocardial infarction: current and emerging applications. J Am Coll Cardiol. 2009;55(1):1–16.
95. Wagner A, et al. Contrast-enhanced MRI and routine single photon emission computed tomography (SPECT) perfusion imaging for detection of subendocardial myocardial infarcts: an imaging study. Lancet. 2003;361(9355):374–9.
96. Thiele H, et al. Reproducibility of chronic and acute infarct size measurement by delayed enhancement-magnetic resonance imaging. J Am Coll Cardiol. 2006;47(8):1641–5.
97. Beek AM, et al. Delayed contrast-enhanced magnetic resonance imaging for the prediction of regional functional improvement after acute myocardial infarction. J Am Coll Cardiol. 2003;42(5):895–901.
98. Gerber BL, et al. Accuracy of contrast-enhanced magnetic resonance imaging in predicting improvement of regional myocardial function in patients after acute myocardial infarction. Circulation. 2002;106(9):1083–9.
99. Kim RJ, et al. The use of contrast-enhanced magnetic resonance imaging to identify reversible myocardial dysfunction. N Engl J Med. 2000;343(20):1445–53.
100. Zhang Q, et al. Artificial intelligence for contrast-free MRI: scar assessment in myocardial infarction using deep learning-based virtual native enhancement. Circulation. 2022;146(20):1492–503.
101. Bhuva AN, et al. A multicenter, scan-rescan, human and machine learning CMR study to test generalizability and precision in imaging biomarker analysis. Circ Cardiovasc Imaging. 2019;12(10):e009214.
102. Wang Y-R, et al. Screening and diagnosis of cardiovascular disease using artificial intelligence-enabled cardiac magnetic resonance imaging. Nat Med. 2024;30(5):1471–80.
103. Kim RJ, et al. Guidelines for training in cardiovascular magnetic resonance (CMR). J Cardiovasc Magn Reson. 2007;9(1):3–4.
104. Fadil H, et al. A deep learning pipeline for automatic analysis of multi-scan cardiovascular magnetic resonance. J Cardiovasc Magn Reson. 2021;23(1):47.
105. Zhang N, et al. Deep learning for diagnosis of chronic myocardial infarction on nonenhanced cardiac cine MRI. Radiology. 2019;291(3):606–17.
106. Pfeiffer MP, Biederman RW. Cardiac MRI: a general overview with emphasis on current use and indications. Med Clin North Am. 2015;99(4):849–61.
107. Larroza A, et al. Texture analysis of cardiac cine magnetic resonance imaging to detect nonviable segments in patients with chronic myocardial infarction. Med Phys. 2018;45(4):1471–80.
108. Baessler B, et al. Subacute and chronic left ventricular myocardial scar: accuracy of texture analysis on nonenhanced cine MR images. Radiology. 2018;286(1):103–12.
109. Jiang B, et al. Development and application of artificial intelligence in cardiac imaging. Br J Radiol. 2020;93(1113):20190812.
110. Upendra RR, Simon R, Linte CA. A deep learning framework for image super-resolution for late gadolinium enhanced cardiac MRI. Comput Cardiol. 2010;2021:48.
111. Bhatia KK, et al. Super-resolution reconstruction of cardiac MRI using coupled dictionary learning. In: IEEE 11th international symposium on Biomedical imaging (ISBI). IEEE; 2014.
112. Ebner M, et al. An automated framework for localization, segmentation and super-resolution reconstruction of fetal brain MRI. NeuroImage. 2020;206:116324.
113. Oktay O, et al. Multi-input cardiac image super-resolution using convolutional neural networks. In: Medical image computing and computer-assisted intervention-MICCAI 2016: 19th international conference, Athens, Greece, October 17–21, 2016, proceedings, part III 19. Springer; 2016.
114. Steeden JA, et al. Rapid whole-heart CMR with single volume super-resolution. J Cardiovasc Magn Reson. 2020;22(1):56.
115. Bustin A, et al. Isotropic reconstruction of MR images using 3D patch-based self-similarity learning. IEEE Trans Med Imaging. 2018;37(8):1932–42.
116. Xiong Z, et al. A global benchmark of algorithms for segmenting the left atrium from late gadolinium-enhanced cardiac magnetic resonance imaging. Med Image Anal. 2021;67:101832.
117. Bernard O, et al. Deep learning techniques for automatic MRI cardiac multi-structures segmentation and diagnosis: is the problem solved? IEEE Trans Med Imaging. 2018;37(11):2514–25.
118. Schuster A, et al. Fully automated cardiac assessment for diagnostic and prognostic stratification following myocardial infarction. J Am Heart Assoc. 2020;9(18):e016612.
119. Hong Q, Zhang C. Multimodal RU-Net: a segmentation network based on multimodal cardiac CMR images. In: 2023 IEEE 9th International Conference on Cloud Computing and Intelligent Systems (CCIS); 2023.
120. Aquaro GD, et al. Diagnostic and prognostic role of late gadolinium enhancement in cardiomyopathies. Eur Heart J Suppl. 2023;25(Suppl C):C130–c136.
121. Fahmy AS, et al. Automated cardiac MR scar quantification in hypertrophic cardiomyopathy using deep

convolutional neural networks. JACC Cardiovasc Imaging. 2018;11(12):1917–8.
122. Leiner T, et al. Machine learning in cardiovascular magnetic resonance: basic concepts and applications. J Cardiovasc Magn Reson. 2019;21(1):61.
123. Chong JH, et al. Artificial intelligence and cardiovascular magnetic resonance imaging in myocardial infarction patients. Curr Probl Cardiol. 2022;47(12):101330.
124. Chen Z, et al. Automatic deep learning-based myocardial infarction segmentation from delayed enhancement MRI. Comput Med Imaging Graph. 2022;95:102014.
125. Kotu LP, et al. Probability mapping of scarred myocardium using texture and intensity features in CMR images. Biomed Eng Online. 2013;12:1–19.
126. Kotu LP, et al. Segmentation of scarred myocardium in cardiac magnetic resonance images. Int Sch Res Notices. 2013;2013(1):504594.
127. Engan K, et al. Exploratory data analysis of image texture and statistical features on myocardium and infarction areas in cardiac magnetic resonance images. In: 2010 annual international conference of the IEEE Engineering in medicine and biology. IEEE; 2010.
128. Larroza A, et al. Differentiation between acute and chronic myocardial infarction by means of texture analysis of late gadolinium enhancement and cine cardiac magnetic resonance imaging. Eur J Radiol. 2017;92:78–83.
129. Zhang Q, et al. Toward replacing late gadolinium enhancement with artificial intelligence virtual native enhancement for gadolinium-free cardiovascular magnetic resonance tissue characterization in hypertrophic cardiomyopathy. Circulation. 2021;144(8):589–99.
130. Keenan NG, et al. Regional variation in cardiovascular magnetic resonance service delivery across the UK. Heart. 2021;107(24):1974–9.
131. Gautam N, et al. Current and future applications of artificial intelligence in coronary artery disease. In: Healthcare. MDPI; 2022.
132. Arnett DK, et al. 2019 ACC/AHA guideline on the primary prevention of cardiovascular disease: a report of the American College of Cardiology/American Heart Association Task Force on Clinical Practice Guidelines. Circulation. 2019;140(11):e596–646.
133. Brautbar A, et al. A genetic risk score based on direct associations with coronary heart disease improves coronary heart disease risk prediction in the atherosclerosis risk in communities (ARIC), but not in the Rotterdam and Framingham offspring. Stud Atherosclerosis. 2012;223(2):421–6.
134. Johri AM, et al. Deep learning artificial intelligence framework for multiclass coronary artery disease prediction using combination of conventional risk factors, carotid ultrasound, and intraplaque neovascularization. Comput Biol Med. 2022;150:106018.
135. Diller GP, et al. Prediction of prognosis in patients with tetralogy of Fallot based on deep learning imaging analysis. Heart. 2020;106(13):1007–14.
136. Slomka PJ, et al. Rationale and design of the REgistry of fast myocardial perfusion imaging with NExt generation SPECT (REFINE SPECT). J Nucl Cardiol. 2020;27(3):1010–21.
137. Cau R, et al. Artificial intelligence in computed tomography plaque characterization: a review. Eur J Radiol. 2021;140:109767.
138. Jie P, et al. Diagnostic value of artificial intelligence-assisted CTA for the assessment of atherosclerosis plaque: a systematic review and meta-analysis. Front Cardiovasc Med. 2024;11:1398963.
139. Choi A, et al. Automated artificial intelligence based interpretation of coronary CTA: plaque volume, plaque characterization and high risk plaque compared with consensus of level III expert readers. J Cardiovasc Comput Tomogr. 2020;14(3):S23.
140. Masuda T, et al. Machine-learning integration of CT histogram analysis to evaluate the composition of atherosclerotic plaques: validation with IB-IVUS. J Cardiovasc Comput Tomogr. 2019;13(2):163–9.
141. Romiti S, et al. Artificial intelligence (AI) and cardiovascular diseases: an unexpected alliance. Cardiol Res Pract. 2020;4972:346.
142. Motwani M, et al. Machine learning for prediction of all-cause mortality in patients with suspected coronary artery disease: a 5-year multicentre prospective registry analysis. Eur Heart J. 2017;38(7):500–7.
143. Javaid A, et al. Medicine 2032: the future of cardiovascular disease prevention with machine learning and digital health technology. Am J Prevent Cardiol. 2022;12:100379.
144. Muscogiuri G, et al. Artificial intelligence in coronary computed tomography angiography: from anatomy to prognosis. Biomed Res Int. 2020;2020(1):6649410.
145. Yoneyama H, et al. Ability of artificial intelligence to diagnose coronary artery stenosis using hybrid images of coronary computed tomography angiography and myocardial perfusion SPECT. Eur J Hybrid Imaging. 2019;3:1–14.
146. van Hamersvelt RW, et al. Deep learning analysis of left ventricular myocardium in CT angiographic intermediate-degree coronary stenosis improves the diagnostic accuracy for identification of functionally significant stenosis. Eur Radiol. 2019;29:2350–9.
147. Arafati A, et al. Artificial intelligence in pediatric and adult congenital cardiac MRI: an unmet clinical need. Cardiovasc Diagn Ther. 2019;9(Suppl 2):S310–s325.
148. Fotaki A, et al. Artificial intelligence in cardiac MRI: is clinical adoption forthcoming? Front Cardiovasc Med. 2022;8

5 AI-Driven Prognostics: Predicting Arrhythmias with CMR Imaging

Amir Ghaffari Jolfayi, Erfan Kohansal, Reza Elahi, Sepehr Jamalkhani, Pevvand Parhizkar, and Golnaz Houshmand

Abstract

Cardiac magnetic resonance (CMR) imaging has emerged as a pivotal tool in evaluating and managing arrhythmia risk across a spectrum of cardiac pathologies, including ischemic heart disease (IHD) and various cardiomyopathies. CMR provides several imaging features, such as the extent and distribution of ventricular scar tissue and atrial fibrosis, as valuable imaging features for guiding clinical decision-making and improving prognosis prediction in patients with cardiac arrhythmias. Recent advancements in Artificial Intelligence (AI) have introduced novel models that leverage CMR data for precise risk stratification and prediction of arrhythmic events. Among the most clinically significant arrhythmias, atrial fibrillation (AF) and ventricular arrhythmias (VAs) have garnered particular attention due to their substantial impact on morbidity and mortality. This chapter explores the pros and cons of different CMR modalities—including late gadolinium enhancement (LGE), T1 and T2 mapping, and four-dimensional (4D) flow imaging—in assessing arrhythmia risk in the context of diverse cardiac diseases. Furthermore, it provides an overview of the progress in AI-driven CMR applications, highlighting their potential to enhance arrhythmia risk assessment and contribute to personalized patient care.

Keywords

Cardiac magnetic resonance imaging · Arrhythmia · Deep learning · Machine learning · Artificial intelligence · Detection · Prognosis

Authors Amir Ghaffari Jolfayi, Erfan Kohansal have contributed equality and shared the first co-authorship.

A. Ghaffari Jolfayi · E. Kohansal · S. Jamalkhani
G. Houshmand (✉)
Cardiovascular Imaging Research Center, Rajaie Cardiovascular Institute, Iran University of Medical Sciences, Tehran, Iran

R. Elahi
Department of Radiology, Zanjan University of Medical Sciences, Zanjan, Iran

P. Parhizkar
School of Medicine, Tehran University of Medical Sciences, Tehran, Iran

5.1 Cardiac MRI in the Assessment of Arrhythmias: Strengths and Limitations

Cardiac arrhythmias encompass a broad spectrum of abnormalities manifesting either as a primary rhythm disorder or as a presentation of an underlying heart disease. They are categorized into three major subgroups: bradyarrhythmias

A. Ghaffari Jolfayi (ed.), *Navigating Cardiology's Future*,
https://doi.org/10.1007/978-981-95-0313-1_5

and heart blocks, supraventricular tachyarrhythmias, and ventricular arrhythmias (VA). Pathologic conditions predisposing to arrhythmia may be congenital or acquired throughout life. Furthermore, inherited abnormalities may be associated with a structurally normal heart or presented as a structural heart disease [1]. Cardiac magnetic resonance (CMR) plays a pivotal role in assessing the risk of arrhythmia incidence during various entities of cardiovascular disorders, and many risk stratification models rely on the CMR parameters for arrhythmia prediction [2–9]. This section reviews the role of CMR in the evaluation and risk stratification of arrhythmia in the context of different entities of cardiovascular diseases, as well as their advantages and drawbacks. In further sections, we also discuss the role of CMR-based AI models in the prediction and risk stratification of arrhythmias and cardiac events.

5.1.1 Ischemic Heart Disease/ Ischemic Cardiomyopathy

Patients with ischemic heart disease (IHD) face a higher risk for the incidence of several types of arrhythmias, either malignant or non-malignant. Nearly half of the deaths among this population are due to sudden cardiac death (SCD), which is attributed to the malignant VAs. The risk is highest during the first month of an acute myocardial infarction (MI) among those with left ventricular dysfunction and/or heart failure [10–12]. Several mechanisms have been proposed to explain the occurrence of VAs in this setting. Myocardial fibrosis is the cornerstone of these mechanisms, which produce re-entry circuits, triggered activity, and abnormal automaticity resulting from peculiar gap junctions and paracrine factors secreted by myofibroblasts [13].

CMR can play a key role in the risk stratification of these patients in several ways. First, CMR is the gold standard modality for measuring left ventricular ejection fraction (LVEF) [14]. The current recommendations for the insertion of an implantable cardioverter defibrillator (ICD) in patients at high risk for malignant VAs and SCD following an acute MI (AMI), despite the suboptimal predictive performance, rely on the post-infarction LVEF values [15–22]. These recommendations are largely based on studies that assessed LVEF using echocardiography [23]. Given the limitations of echocardiography—particularly in patients with poor acoustic windows and its reliance on 2D assumptions rather than true 3D volumetric assessment—cardiac magnetic resonance (CMR) offers a more accurate measurement of left ventricular ejection fraction (LVEF). Utilizing CMR for LVEF assessment may enhance risk stratification and improve decision-making for ICD implantation, thereby aiding in the prevention of arrhythmias and sudden cardiac death in this population. Second, CMR can detect myocardial fibrosis with high precision via a contrast-based method delineating late gadolinium enhancement (LGE) [24, 25]. The presence, extent, and pattern of the LGE are strongly associated with the incidence of malignant VAs, adverse cardiovascular events, and mortality in patients with IHD or among those who are candidates for possible ICD insertion [26–30]. More importantly, the LGE gray zone (i.e., a myocardium with a signal intensity within the range of 35% to 50% of the maximal signal intensity) as indicators of the peri-infarct zone with a heterogeneous tissue mixture of the viable myocardium and replacement fibrosis, is among of the strongest predictors for the incidence of serious VAs in patients with previous MI and/or ischemic cardiomyopathy (ICM), with a larger extent of the LGE gray zone delineates a higher risk of arrhythmia [26, 31–33].

LV entropy, which is directly calculated from the probability distribution of the signal intensity of the LV myocardium pixels on LGE images, is correlated with all-cause death independently, VAs requiring therapy, or hospitalization due to heart failure [34]. Moreover, in a prospective cohort of 162 patients with AMI, a larger extent of penumbra area in the CMR (defined as a myocardial area with an LGE signal intensity of 25–50% of maximal signal intensity) was associated with an increased risk for the occurrence of ventricular tachycardia (VT) in the subacute phase [35]. Ultimately, tissue characterization utilized in CMR mapping enables the delineation of small variations in the tissue structures and components. T1 mapping before and after gadolinium administration enables better discrimination of interstitial fibrosis and normal myocardium by calculating the extracellular volume (ECV) fraction [36].

5.1.2 Non-ischemic Dilated Cardiomyopathy/Myocarditis

Patients with non-ischemic dilated cardiomyopathy (NIDCM) may experience VT as the initial manifestation of their disease or later during the course of the cardiomyopathy, imposing a great risk for syncope and SCD [37]. Both the DANISH and DEFINITE trials showed that prophylactic ICD therapy significantly reduces sudden cardiac death in patients with NIDCM, although neither trial demonstrated a statistically significant reduction in all-cause mortality [38, 39]. CMR may augment the risk stratification for the incidence of VA among patients with NIDCM in several ways. The presence of LGE in the CMR of patients with NIDCM has been linked to a nearly fourfold increased odds of experiencing serious VAs, and when considered along with the LVEF, has been found to yield its risk stratification properties [6, 40]. Likewise, in patients with NIDCM, LV gray zone and entropy are implicated as correlated with the incidence of VAs [34, 41]. The use of the presence and extent of myocardial fibrosis, detected by cardiac MRI, to guide decisions regarding ICD implantation in this population is an area of active and ongoing research [42]. ECV fraction has been the subject of several recent studies as a non-invasive tool for assessing the risk of arrhythmic events among patients with NIDCM. Several studies have delineated that ECV fraction is a strong independent predictor of the incidence of arrhythmia during NIDCM, and several cutoffs have been proposed for this purpose [43, 44].

Another CMR tool that indicates the risk for adverse cardiovascular events in the future among patients with NIDCM is the T1 mapping. A prospective prognosis study revealed that T1 mapping, as a measure of diffuse myocardial interstitial fibrosis, can independently predict the risk of all-cause death and heart failure (HF) [45]. It was demonstrated that a T1 Z-score has been suggested as an independent predictor of arrhythmic events' incidence [43]. In a more recent study evaluating the role of CMR parameters in the prediction of the risk of adverse events in patients with NIDCM, T1 values and ECV fraction were found to be strongly associated with the incidence of the secondary composite outcome of HF hospitalization, incidence of VAs, and insertion of ICD and/or cardiac resynchronization therapy. However, on the multi-variable analysis with adjustment for LVEF and New York Heart Association class, the maximum value of the native T1 failed to efficiently demonstrate predictive capability for the incidence of this secondary composite outcome. In contrast, the mean value of the ECV fraction remained an independent predictor of the outcome [46]. Ultimately, a recent systematic review and meta-analysis concluded that higher ECV fraction and native T1 values are associated with a higher risk for morbidity and mortality in patients with NIDCM [47].

5.1.3 Other Forms of Cardiomyopathy

Hypertrophic cardiomyopathy (HCM), arrhythmogenic cardiomyopathy (ACM), and left ventricular non-compaction cardiomyopathy (LVNC) are susceptible to the incidence of arrhythmias [1, 48–54]. The American Heart Association (AHA) and the American College of Cardiology guidelines recommend that patients with HCM undergo risk stratification for sudden cardiac death (SCD) at diagnosis and at regular intervals thereafter. A major component in the recommended model for risk stratification is left ventricular septum diameter (LVSD), in which a diameter of ≥30 millimeters has been considered a risk factor for the incidence of malignant VAs and SCD [55, 56].

CMR can help classify the risk of SCD in patients with HCM in several ways other than those previously mentioned for other disease entities. First, CMR is the gold standard imaging modality for the anatomic evaluation of the heart and quantification of ventricular size and function [57]. Structural parameters potentially affecting the risk of SCD and malignant VAs are higher left ventricular wall thickness and presence of apical aneurysm [58], which can be better visualized in CMR. A remarkable left ventricular outlet (LVOT) obstruction has been linked to a higher risk for the incidence of SCD or ICD discharge occurrence [58, 59], although LVOT gradients are best assessed by echo, 4-dimensional flow CMR has emerged as a non-invasive tool for assessing and quantifying flow parameters, enabling the CMR to calculate pressure gradients accurately [58, 59]. More importantly, LGE, as an indicator of myocardial fibrosis, has been assumed to be correlated with the incidence of non-sustained VT in the Holter monitoring of patients with HCM [60]. Furthermore, among patients with HCM, extensive LGE, assumed as the involvement of $\geq$15% of the left ventricular mass, is a predictor for the incidence of SCD, and every increase in the extent of the LGE is responsible for a higher risk for SCD [61, 62].

As a pivotal tool for diagnosing ACM, CMR can also help in risk stratification of affected patients by providing invaluable information on biventricular structure, function, and the extent of fibro-adipose infiltration. In this regard, the severity of left or right ventricular dysfunction reflects the risk for incidence of SCD [63]. Additionally, patients with isolated left ventricular involvement, exhibiting systolic dysfunction and/or fibro-adipose infiltration on their CMR imaging, demonstrate the worst prognosis for aborted cardiac arrest or sudden cardiac death (SCD), making them suitable candidates for an implantable cardioverter-defibrillator (ICD) [64]. Hence, the new diagnostic criteria of ACM mandate the assessment of LGE extent within both the left and right ventricles as an indicator of fibro-adipose infiltration [65]. For patients with LVNC, CMR is an ideal and comprehensive tool for risk stratification regarding the incidence of adverse cardiovascular outcomes, including arrhythmias [66].

In patients with LVNC, left ventricular dilation, dysfunction, and/or LGE observed on CMR imaging significantly elevate the risk of adverse cardiac events, including ventricular arrhythmias and cardiac death [67, 68]. In addition, a compacted myocardial thinning, as portrayed by the long-axis steady-state free precession CMR cine images, is associated with an increased risk of adverse cardiovascular outcomes [69]. Ultimately, the exploitation of comprehensive CMR provides various parameters with significant implications on the incidence of adverse cardiovascular events, including VAs. In this regard, CMR-based risk prediction models, using multiple CMR parameters, have been proposed to predict the risk of developing adverse cardiovascular outcomes of LVNC [70]. Given the phenotypic overlap with dilated cardiomyopathy (DCM) and ischemic cardiomyopathy (ICM), risk stratification strategies applied in DCM may be partially extrapolated to LVNC patients, particularly in those with reduced ejection fraction and myocardial fibrosis [71].

Despite all the benefits of CMR, it carries several relative drawbacks. First, CMR is not applicable in patients with some specific metallic devices, and evaluation of the fibrosis needs administration of contrast, which potentially restricts its use in patients with severe renal failure. Second, some of the parameters above are time-consuming to assess, are susceptible to errors, and the available data on their prognostic significance are limited or inclined to bias. Furthermore, the assessment of some parameters (e.g., LVEF) is operator-dependent and accompanied by inter-observer variability. Eventually, tissue characterization and myocardial mapping need expertise, as they are not widely used and lack unified cut-offs for risk stratification. Hence, to delineate the role of CMR in clinical practice as a tool for assessing the risk of future arrhythmic events, its capabilities must be investigated through adequately powered RCTs with long-term follow-ups [13, 72, 73].

5.2 CMR-Based Risk Stratification for Ventricular Arrhythmias: AI Insights

SCD, followed by life-threatening VAs with societal and personal impacts, is a devastating event that affects 50–100 per 100,000 individuals each year [74]. VAs encompass a variety of cardiac disorders, including premature ventricular contractions, VT, and VF. VAs significantly contribute to the burden of cardiovascular diseases (CVDs) as a leading cause of global morbidity and mortality, emphasizing the requirement for effective diagnosis, treatment, and prevention strategies to manage and reduce the risks associated with these arrhythmias [75].

Some known key risk factors for VAs include structural cardiac disorders, prior MI, obesity, diabetes, hypertension, and smoking. Although progress has been made in discovering these related factors, VA occurrence remains unpredictable. This underscores the necessity of identifying other risk factors to improve risk stratification and allow for more targeted interventions to reduce the incidence of VAs [76]. On the other hand, many SCD events happen suddenly in individuals who were not previously detected as high-risk, largely because of the limitations of present risk stratification strategies, revealing the importance of developed risk stratification strategies for VAs [77].

AI tools are increasingly being employed to address complicated medical challenges, particularly in electrophysiology. By utilizing extensive and detailed datasets, AI-related prediction models have shown the capacity to improve the risk stratification of VAs. The use of Machine Learning (ML) with intracardiac electrograms from implantable cardioverter-defibrillators (ICDs) [78], employing variational mode decomposition (VMD)-based features along with the C4.5 classifier for detecting VAs [79], and the CatBoost model to predict long-term VAs [80], are some examples of the effectiveness of AI for risk stratification in VAs. On the other hand, ML techniques for reconstructing MRI data are gaining significant attention in research, and various methods are being provided for performing these reconstructions. These advanced techniques offer innovative approaches to improve the quality and efficiency of MRI data processing, enhancing the potential for more accurate and detailed imaging outcomes [81].

A more comprehensive risk assessment than traditional methods, considering VAs and SCD, can be obtained using advanced imaging techniques and detailed clinical information. As an example, Popescu et al. conducted a study to develop a Deep Learning (DL) model aimed at SCD within 10 years, utilizing CMR images alongside clinical data from 156 individuals with ischemic heart disease. Among these participants, 41 experienced SCD events. The model underwent external validation with a separate cohort of 113 patients, 22 of whom had SCD events. The model obtained an AUC of 0.87 for the internal and 0.72 for the external datasets, with 10-year integrated Brier scores of 0.12 and 0.14, respectively. This method, which combines cardiac imaging with clinical data to predict SCD, holds promise for enhancing predictive accuracy and improving patient outcomes [82].

Another study also provided a novel DL approach, combining neural networks with survival analysis, for predicting patient-specific survival curves from contrast-enhanced cardiac MRI and clinical data in IHD patients. The SSCAR approach includes two neural networks: a 3D convolutional network from unsegmented LGE-CMR images and a fully connected network processing clinical data. SSCAR's patient-specific survival curves provide enhanced predictions of SCD risk over 10 years, showing potential to improve clinical decision-making on multi-center internal validation and an independent test set; the model achieved concordance indexes of 0.83 and 0.74, with 10-year integrated Brier scores of 0.12 and 0.14. Using only raw cardiac images, the DL model outperformed standard survival models based on clinical data alone [82].

Another study highlighted the role of MRI data, particularly CMR, in improving VA risk stratification in patients with acute myocarditis (AM) through ML models. The study found that certain CMR variables, including LGE patterns and T2-hyper signal, were crucial in predicting major adverse cardiovascular events (MACE), including VAs. The researchers developed an ML model using CMR data, outperforming traditional statistical methods like logistic regression in predicting MACE. Specifically, the Random Forest ML model, which incorporated clinical, biological, and CMR data, showed superior accuracy, with an AUC of 0.74 compared to 0.70 for traditional methods. The model was also validated in an external cohort, maintaining strong predictive performance (AUC of 0.73). In conclusion, the study demonstrated that incorporating CMR imaging with ML models significantly enhances the ability to predict VAs and other cardiac events in AM patients, providing a more reliable risk stratification tool than traditional approaches [83].

The improved predictive capability of the ML model, particularly using image data, highlights its potential to offer more accurate risk assessments for SCD, potentially leading to better-informed clinical decisions and more personalized patient management. Smole et al. trained an ML model for predicting the 5-year SCD risk in 2302 individuals with HCM using multiple variables. These variables included imaging data besides demographics, physical exams, genetics, and medications. The model obtained an AUC of 0.70 for predicting SCD, outperforming a previous SCD risk assessment tool for HCM, which had an AUC of 0.63 [84]. O'Mahony et al. also aimed to evaluate the diagnostic potential of ML-related texture characteristic analysis of LGE images from cardiac MRI in identifying VT in HCM patients. Among the 64 patients studied, 21 (32.8%) had VT. Of the eight ML models tested, the KNN model with SMOTE showed the highest diagnostic accuracy in detecting VT. It correctly identified 40 out of 42 (95.2%) VT-positive cases and 40 out of 43 (93.0%) VT-negative cases, with a sensitivity of 95.2%, specificity of 93.0%, and overall accuracy of 94.1. Moreover, ML-based texture analysis of LGE areas appears to be a favorable strategy for distinguishing HCM individuals with/without VT [85].

In another study, a deep learning model (LVM-AI) was applied to 12-lead ECGs to predict left ventricular mass, aiming to improve the detection of left ventricular hypertrophy (LVH) compared to traditional ECG methods. The model was trained and tested on data from large cohorts, showing a strong correlation with CMR-derived LV mass and better or comparable LVH discrimination compared to traditional ECG rules. Additionally, LVM-AI-predicted LVH was linked to a greater risk of cardiovascular events, including VAs. The findings underscore how DL-enhanced ECG predictions can improve risk stratification by aligning with MRI data and providing precise myocardial characteristics imaging. This combined approach helps detect individuals at higher risk for VAs, refining cardiovascular risk assessment and enabling more targeted interventions [86].

Another study by Akyea et al. examined cardiac MRI data in conjunction with unsupervised ML to enhance risk stratification for VAs in individuals with mitral valve prolapse (MVP) without prominent mitral regurgitation or LV dysfunction. The study employed a data-driven hierarchical k-means algorithm to detect phenotypic clusters among 474 MVP patients based on cardiac MRI findings, including LGE, which detects myocardial fibrosis. The analysis revealed two distinct clusters. Herein, Cluster 2 patients who exhibited more severe mitral valve degeneration, chamber remodeling, and myocardial fibrosis, as seen on LGE-MRI, had a significantly higher risk of developing arrhythmic events such as sustained VT, SCD, or unexplained syncope. The increased risk was notable even after adjusting for LGE extent, with a hazard ratio of 3.79 compared to cluster 1. This study highlights the potential of MRI-based imaging phenotyping combined with ML to better predict arrhythmic risk in MVP patients. This approach emphasizes the importance of detailed imaging data for personalized risk assessment in this patient population [87].

The efficacy of implantable ICDs in preventing SCD in non-ischemic cardiomyopathy patients is under debate. Advancements in AI-related strategies have provided a promising tool for addressing this issue. AI can analyze complex datasets, including cardiac MRI images, to offer more accurate risk assessments in identifying prognostic accuracy for VAs in non-ischemic systolic heart failure patients before ICD implantation. One such innovation is the development of the DEEP RISK model, a multi-modal DL approach designed to predict arrhythmic risk by integrating LGE cardiac MRI, ECG, and clinical data of patients. The DEEP RISK model was developed to predict arrhythmia risk in 289 patients before ICD implantation. Employing a residual variational AE to derive physiological features from LGE-MRI and ECG, DEEP RISK predicted malignant VAs with an AUC of 0.84, sensitivity of 0.98, and specificity of 0.73 in the validation cohort. Models trained on individual modalities had lower AUROC values (MRI: 0.80, ECG: 0.54, Clinical: 0.64), highlighting the superiority of the multimodal approach [88].

On the other hand, there is also a critical requirement for advanced methods in the automatic segmentation and quantification of cardiac fibrosis, besides enhanced risk stratification for SCD. Many individuals at higher risk for VA and SCD who receive an ICD may not always receive the appropriate therapy from the device. Fibrosis identified on LGE-CMR is known to be linked with a higher VA risk. The study by Lieshout et al. introduced a novel two-stage DL network designed to segment the left ventricular myocardium and fibrosis from LGE-CMR images. Additionally, it aimed to enhance the prediction of ICD therapy needs using a graph neural network (GNN) that integrates features from both the myocardium and fibrosis, along with the left ventricular geometry. The segmentation network demonstrated superior performance to prior state-of-the-art methods on 2D CMR data, achieving Dice scores of 0.82 and 0.77 for myocardium and fibrosis segmentation, respectively. The ICD therapy prediction network, which relies on CMR data, achieved an AUC of 0.60 and outperformed existing baseline methods related to the present guidelines for ICD implantation. This work provided a considerable foundation for further investigation to improve risk stratification for VA and SCD [89]. On the other side, improved models to detect patients at a decreased risk of VA are essential for ICD candidates to reduce the potential for ICD-associated events and to optimize the use of these devices. Krebs et al. conducted the CERTAINTY study using DL to predict VA based on cine CMR imaging to address this need. Two neural networks were developed in 350 ICD recipients (178 with ischemic cardiomyopathy) who had undergone CMR before ICD implantation. The Cine Fingerprint Extractor autonomously captures structure/function characteristics from cine CMR, creating a "cine fingerprint." The Risk Predictor uses this fingerprint to generate a risk score for predicting outcomes. In this study, individuals who experienced VA (n = 96) had a significantly greater risk score compared to those who did not. The cine risk score remained correlated with VA even after adjusting for clinical factors, cardiac structure, and CMR-related scar extent. The results suggest that cine CMR inherently captures features that can enhance VA risk prediction in primary prevention ICD candidates [90].

5.3 CMR Value for the Approach to AF: Predicting AF and the Use of Different Sequences in CMR

To understand the potential of AI-enhanced MRI for AF prediction, it is essential first to consider the underlying pathophysiological processes. Structural and functional changes in the left atrium (LA) often precede the development of AF and contribute to its initiation and maintenance. These changes, collectively called atrial remodeling, include LA enlargement, decreased LA function, fibrosis and scarring, electrical remodeling, and autonomic remodeling [91]. LA enlargement is one of the most consistent findings associated with AF, reflecting the cumulative effect of various cardiovascular stressors, and is a strong predictor of AF development. Atrial fibrosis is a hallmark of structural remodeling in AF, with the accumulation of extracellular matrix proteins leading to electrical uncoupling of cardiomyocytes, creating a substrate for re-entry and promoting AF [91]. CMR has emerged as a powerful tool for assessing these changes due to its excellent spatial resolution, tissue characterization capabilities, and ability to comprehensively evaluate cardiac structure and function without ionizing radiation [91]. Here, we first overview CMR techniques developed to evaluate atrial remodeling. Then, we discuss the role of AI-based CMR analysis techniques for AF prediction and risk stratification.

5.3.1 Cine CMR

Cine CMR provides accurate measurements of LA volumes and allows the calculation of various LA functional indices [92]. Cine CMR offers superior spatial resolution compared to echocardiography, particularly for the LA, which can be challenging to image completely with ultrasound due to its posterior location [93].

5.3.2 Real-Time CMR

This dynamic evaluation is particularly relevant for AF detection because it can reveal abnormalities in atrial performance that may not be apparent during static imaging [94]. For instance, real-time CMR can demonstrate impaired atrial reservoir, conduit, or booster pump functions, often compromised in patients at risk of AF [95]. Real-time CMR can detect subtle irregularities in atrial contraction and relaxation by capturing rapid changes in atrial size, shape, and function throughout the cardiac cycle and under different loading conditions [94]. These irregularities might indicate underlying electrical or structural abnormalities predisposing to AF. Moreover, real-time CMR can potentially capture paroxysmal AF episodes during imaging, providing direct evidence of the arrhythmia [94].

5.3.3 Feature-Tracking CMR

Feature-tracking CMR enables assessing LA phasic function by tracking myocardial deformation throughout the cardiac cycle [96]. Feature-tracking algorithms analyze the motion of myocardial tissue voxels on standard cine CMR images without additional tagged sequences [96, 97]. Key parameters derived from feature-tracking include LA volumes (maximum, minimum, pre-atrial contraction), LA emptying fractions (total, passive, active), peak LA longitudinal strain, and LA strain rate [96]. Habibi et al. used feature-tracking CMR to investigate the association between LA function and incident AF in the Multi-Ethnic Study of Atherosclerosis (MESA) [98]. They found that decreased passive and total LA emptying fractions and reduced peak LA strain were independently associated with new-onset AF. This study demonstrated the potential of CMR-derived functional parameters for AF risk stratification in an asymptomatic population [98].

5.3.4 Late Gadolinium Enhancement (LGE) MRI

LGE-MRI allows visualization and quantification of atrial fibrosis [99]. After administering a gadolinium-based contrast agent, fibrotic areas appear hyperenhanced due to increased extracellular space and delayed contrast washout. The degree of enhancement on LGE images correlates with the extent of fibrosis [99]. Studies have shown that areas with higher LGE intensity are associated with lower voltage and slower conduction velocity in the atrial wall, which are markers of an arrhythmogenic substrate [99]. Caixal et al. demonstrated the accuracy of LGE-MRI in identifying left atrial arrhythmogenic substrate by analyzing voltage and conduction velocity at the areas of LGE [99]. They found a significant negative correlation between LGE with voltage ($r = 0.39$, $P < 0.001$) and conduction velocity ($r = 0.25$, $P < 0.001$) [99]. Quantification of LGE has traditionally relied on manual segmentation, which is time-consuming and subject to inter-observer variability [99].

5.3.5 High-Resolution 3D LGE Imaging

High-resolution 3D LGE imaging is increasingly recognized as a valuable tool in the management of AF, particularly for guiding catheter ablation procedures. Recent studies have reinforced its clinical relevance by demonstrating its ability to noninvasively visualize atrial fibrosis and structural remodeling. In Letsas et al. study, 3D LGE-CMR significantly enhanced substrate mapping by clearly delineating regions of atrial fibrosis, enabling more targeted and effective ablation strategies. This imaging approach was associated with improved procedural precision and potential for better long-term arrhythmia control [100]. Similarly, Nyktari et al. showed that 3D LGE-CMR provides comprehensive insights into left atrial structural changes, including fibrosis extent, wall thinning, and volumetric alterations [101]. These features have prognostic value and can aid in identifying patients at higher risk for recurrence post-ablation. Together, these findings support the integration of 3D LGE-CMR into AF ablation workflows, offering a more personalized and anatomically informed approach to treatment planning [100, 101].

5.3.6 T1 Mapping

T1 mapping quantifies myocardial T1 relaxation times, which reflect tissue composition [102]. This method provides valuable information through parameters such as native T1 and ECV, enabling the detection of subtle tissue changes that might not be apparent in conventional imaging [102]. While most studies have focused on ventricular T1 mapping, emerging research explores its utility in atrial tissue characterization and AF prediction [102].

5.3.7 4D Flow MRI

An innovative technique that allows for the visualization and quantification of blood flow patterns within the atria [103]. This method provides insights into atrial hemodynamics and can identify abnormal flow patterns associated with remodeling, offering a unique perspective on the functional consequences of structural changes [103]. In the context of AF detection, 4D Flow MRI can reveal abnormal flow patterns such as vortex formation, stasis, or turbulence within the left atrium [103, 104]. These flow disturbances are often associated with structural remodeling and can predispose to thrombus formation, a major complication of AF [104]. Additionally, 4D Flow MRI can quantify parameters like flow velocity, kinetic energy, and vorticity, which may be altered in patients prone to AF [104]. By identifying these hemodynamic changes, 4D Flow MRI can potentially detect early signs of atrial dysfunction before the onset of sustained AF, making it a valuable tool for risk stratification and early intervention [105].

5.3.8 Black-Blood Imaging

This method suppresses the signal from flowing blood, allowing for enhanced visualization of the atrial walls, and is particularly useful for detecting AF-related changes in atrial structure. In the context of AF detection, black-blood imaging can reveal areas of wall thickening, which may indicate fibrosis or inflammation associated with AF [106–108]. It can also clearly delineate the pulmonary vein ostia and left atrial appendage, areas often involved in AF initiation and propagation [106]. By providing clear images of the atrial walls, this technique can detect subtle structural abnormalities that may predispose to AF, such as crypts, diverticula, or areas of wall thinning. These structural irregularities can create regions of conduction heterogeneity, potentially serving as substrates for AF initiation or maintenance [109].

5.3.9 First-Pass Perfusion Imaging

While traditionally used for ventricular assessment, this technique can provide valuable information about atrial perfusion. In the context of

AF detection, first-pass perfusion imaging can reveal microvascular dysfunction in the atrial myocardium [110]. Impaired atrial perfusion may contribute to atrial fibrosis and electrical remodeling, key factors in AF development [110]. By identifying areas of reduced perfusion or perfusion heterogeneity in the atria, this technique can detect early signs of atrial ischemia or other perfusion abnormalities that may predispose to AF [111]. Additionally, perfusion imaging might reveal underlying coronary artery disease affecting atrial branches, which could be a contributing factor to AF in some patients [111].

5.4 CMR-Based Risk Stratification for AF: AI Insights

Machine learning (ML) techniques have recently been applied to analyze cardiac MRI data for AF prediction. Support Vector Machine (SVM) has been a popular choice, demonstrating good performance in discriminating AF cases from controls. Pujadas et al. and Dykstra et al. utilized SVM in their studies, highlighting its effectiveness in handling high-dimensional data and its robust theoretical foundations [112, 113]. Pujadas et al. used SVM for their hierarchical models, extracting 262 radiomics features from each CMR study, including 26 LV shape features, 26 RV shape features, 26 LV myocardium shape features, 36 LV myocardium first-order features, and 148 LV myocardium texture features. Their best-performing model for AF prediction achieved an accuracy of 0.71 and an AUC of 0.76 [113].

Random Survival Forests (RSF) have also shown promise, particularly in predicting new-onset AF [114]. Dykstra et al. found that RSF models outperformed traditional Cox proportional-hazard models, showcasing the ability of ensemble methods to capture complex interactions between variables. They employed RSF models using 115 variables from three data domains: CMR-based disease phenotype, patient health questionnaire, and electronic health records. Their RSF-based model (CIROC-AF-20) using the top 20 variables achieved an overall C-index of 0.78 for predicting new-onset AF, with time-dependent AUCs of 0.80, 0.79, and 0.78 at 1-, 2-, and 3-years, respectively [112].

Logistic Regression (LR) remains widely used, especially for predicting AF recurrence after catheter ablation. Fan et al.'s meta-analysis revealed that 60% of studies employed LR, likely due to its interpretability and well-established statistical properties. The pooled C-index for LR models was 0.785 (95% CI 0.737 to 0.833) in the training set and 0.804 (95% CI 0.735 to 0.872) in the validation set [115].

Other ML algorithms explored in various studies include K-nearest neighbor (KNN), Cox proportional hazard model (COX), adaptive boosting (AdaBoost), artificial neural networks (ANN), extreme gradient boosting (XGBoost), random forest (RF), and decision trees (DT). This diversity of approaches reflects the ongoing search for optimal predictive models in AF research [115].

Deep learning (DL), as a subset of ML, uses multilayer neural networks to extract high-dimensional features and learn from the data in a task-oriented manner. There are various DL networks developed for classification and prediction tasks, including Convolutional Neural Networks (CNNs), deep neural networks (DNNs), Autoencoders (AEs), recurrent neural networks (RNNs), dual path networks (DPNs), generative adversarial networks (GANs), etc. [116, 117]. In the context of AF prediction, DL models have demonstrated superior performance in some studies compared to ML models. Fan et al. reported that compared to other methods, CNN models achieved the highest C-index, specificity, and sensitivity in predicting AF, underlining the potential of DL approaches in extracting relevant features from imaging data. The overall pooled C-index for CNN models was 0.862 in the training and 0.861 in the validation set [115].

Regarding MR modalities and features, most studies relied on cine MRI using balanced steady-state free precession (bSSFP) sequences to acquire short-axis and long-axis heart images. These sequences provide excellent contrast between blood and myocardium, allowing for accurate assessment of cardiac structure and function. LGE imaging has been incorporated in some studies to evaluate myocardial fibrosis, which may play a role in the pathogenesis of AF [113].

LA volume, particularly when indexed to body surface area (LAVi), has consistently emerged as a strong predictor of AF across multiple studies. This aligns with the understanding that LA remodeling is a key factor in AF development and progression [113, 118]. In Pujadas et al.'s study, LA volume ranked first in feature importance [113]. Ventricular parameters have also proven valuable, with left ventricular end-diastolic volume (LVEDV), end-systolic volume (LVESV), LVEF, and mass (LVM) commonly included in predictive models [113]. Pujadas et al. found that LVM alone had higher accuracy in all models than LVSV. Some studies have considered right ventricular measurements, recognizing the potential role of right-sided cardiac remodeling in AF pathophysiology [113].

A significant advancement in the field has been the incorporation of radiomics features extracted from MR images. These features provide a more detailed cardiac structure and tissue composition characterization beyond conventional metrics. Shape features, such as maximum 2D and 3D diameters, surface area, and sphericity, have shown discriminative power in AF prediction [113, 118, 119]. First-order features like energy, median, mean, and root mean squared values offer insights into the distribution of signal intensities within an ROI. Texture features, including grey-level non-uniformity, coarseness, contrast, and entropy, capture patterns of tissue heterogeneity that may reflect underlying pathological changes [113].

The importance of specific radiomics features varies across studies and AF outcomes. For instance, Pujadas et al. found that shape features depicting the "maximum diameter" presented the most discriminative power in AF prediction alongside texture features of non-uniformity. In heart failure models, shape features related to chamber dimensions and elongation (e.g., minor axis) provided additional predictive value. For myocardial infarction, texture features such as coarseness and large area emphasis were more prominent [113].

ML models incorporating radiomics features generally outperformed those using only clinical characteristics or standard CMR indices. Thus, combining vascular risk factors, conventional CMR metrics, and radiomics features is expected to yield the best predictive performance for AF. It is worth noting that while these AI-enhanced MRI techniques show great promise, challenges remain in standardizing radiomics feature extraction and ensuring reproducibility across different centers and MRI scanners. Additionally, the clinical implementation of these advanced techniques requires careful consideration of workflow integration and the interpretability of complex machine learning models.

5.5 Conclusion

In this chapter, we have discussed the transformative role of AI models in leveraging CMR data to predict arrhythmias and rhythm abnormalities. AI-based models have shown great promise in enhancing the precision of risk stratification, enabling earlier interventions and personalized treatment options for conditions such as AF and VAs. Advancements in MRI techniques, including LGE, T1 and T2 mapping, and 4D flow imaging, have provided detailed insights into myocardial and atrial tissue characteristics. By integrating these complex imaging features, AI algorithms can identify subtle patterns and predictors of arrhythmia risk that may not be visible through conventional analysis. Despite these achievements, challenges such as the need for larger, diverse datasets, improved standardization of imaging protocols, and validation of AI models across clinical settings remain. Addressing these limitations will translate AI innovations into widespread clinical patient care.

References

1. Wilde AAM, et al. European heart rhythm association (EHRA)/Heart Rhythm Society (HRS)/ Asia Pacific Heart Rhythm Society (APHRS)/ Latin American Heart Rhythm Society (LAHRS) expert consensus statement on the state of genetic testing for cardiac diseases. Heart Rhythm. 2022;19(7):e1–e60.
2. Zaman S, Kovoor P. Sudden cardiac death early after myocardial infarction. Circulation. 2014;129(23):2426–35.
3. Deyell MW, Krahn AD, Goldberger JJ. Sudden cardiac death risk stratification. Circ Res. 2015;116(12):1907–18.
4. Mavrogeni S, et al. Prediction of ventricular arrhythmias using cardiovascular magnetic resonance. Eur Heart J Cardiovasc Imaging. 2013;14(6):518–25.
5. Dawson DK, et al. Prognostic role of CMR in patients presenting with ventricular arrhythmias. JACC Cardiovasc Imaging. 2013;6(3):335–44.
6. Marco AD, et al. Improved risk stratification for ventricular arrhythmias and sudden death in patients with nonischemic dilated cardiomyopathy. J Am Coll Cardiol. 2021;77(23):2890–905.
7. Guglielmo M, Pontone G. Risk stratification in cardiomyopathies (dilated, hypertrophic, and arrhythmogenic cardiomyopathy) by cardiac magnetic resonance imaging. Eur Heart J Suppl. 2021;23(Suppl E):E118–22.
8. Nazarian S, Lima JAC. Cardiovascular Magnetic Resonance for Risk Stratification of Arrhythmia in Hypertrophic Cardiomyopathy. J Am Coll Cardiol. 2008;51(14):1375–6.
9. Arevalo HJ, et al. Arrhythmia risk stratification of patients after myocardial infarction using personalized heart models. Nat Commun. 2016;7(1):11437.
10. Berg DD, et al. Modes and timing of death in 66 252 patients with non-ST-segment elevation acute coronary syndromes enrolled in 14 TIMI trials. Eur Heart J. 2018;39(42):3810–20.
11. Grey C, et al. One in four major ischaemic heart disease events are fatal and 60% are pre-hospital deaths: a national data-linkage study (ANZACS-QI 8). Eur Heart J. 2015;38(3):172–80.
12. Solomon SD, et al. Sudden death in patients with myocardial infarction and left ventricular dysfunction, heart failure, or both. N Engl J Med. 2005;352(25):2581–8.
13. Gräni C, et al. Sudden cardiac death in ischemic heart disease: from imaging arrhythmogenic substrate to guiding therapies. JACC Cardiovasc Imaging. 2020;13(10):2223–38.
14. Grothues F, et al. Comparison of interstudy reproducibility of cardiovascular magnetic resonance with two-dimensional echocardiography in normal subjects and in patients with heart failure or left ventricular hypertrophy. Am J Cardiol. 2002;90(1):29–34.
15. Kusumoto FM, et al. HRS/ACC/AHA expert consensus statement on the use of implantable cardioverter-defibrillator therapy in patients who are not included or not well represented in clinical trials. Circulation. 2014;130(1):94–125.
16. Zeppenfeld K, et al. 2022 ESC guidelines for the management of patients with ventricular arrhythmias and the prevention of sudden cardiac death: developed by the task force for the management of patients with ventricular arrhythmias and the prevention of sudden cardiac death of the European Society of Cardiology (ESC) endorsed by the Association for European Paediatric and Congenital Cardiology (AEPC). Eur Heart J. 2022;43(40):3997–4126.
17. Moss AJ, et al. Prophylactic implantation of a defibrillator in patients with myocardial infarction and reduced ejection fraction. N Engl J Med. 2002;346(12):877–83.
18. Moss AJ, et al. Improved survival with an implanted defibrillator in patients with coronary disease at high risk for ventricular arrhythmia. N Engl J Med. 1996;335(26):1933–40.
19. Bigger JT. Prophylactic use of implanted cardiac defibrillators in patients at high risk for ventricular arrhythmias after coronary-artery bypass graft surgery. N Engl J Med. 1997;337(22):1569–75.
20. Buxton AE, et al. Electrophysiologic testing to identify patients with coronary artery disease who are at risk for sudden death. N Engl J Med. 2000;342(26):1937–45.
21. Hohnloser SH, et al. Prophylactic use of an implantable cardioverter–defibrillator after acute myocardial infarction. N Engl J Med. 2004;351(24):2481–8.
22. Bardy GH, et al. Amiodarone or an implantable cardioverter–defibrillator for congestive heart failure. N Engl J Med. 2005;352(3):225–37.
23. de Haan S, et al. Assessment of left ventricular ejection fraction in patients eligible for ICD therapy: discrepancy between cardiac magnetic resonance imaging and 2D echocardiography. Neth Hear J. 2014;22(10):449–55.
24. Iles LM, et al. Histological validation of cardiac magnetic resonance analysis of regional and diffuse interstitial myocardial fibrosis. Eur Heart J Cardiovasc Imaging. 2014;16(1):14–22.
25. GhaffariJolfayi A, et al. Machine learning-based interpretation of non-contrast feature tracking strain analysis and T1/T2 mapping for assessing myocardial viability. Sci Rep. 2025;15(1):753.
26. Disertori M, et al. Myocardial fibrosis assessment by LGE is a powerful predictor of ventricular Tachyarrhythmias in ischemic and nonischemic LV dysfunction. JACC Cardiovasc Imaging. 2016;9(9):1046–55.
27. Scott PA, et al. Left ventricular scar burden specifies the potential for ventricular arrhythmogenesis: an LGE-CMR study. J Cardiovasc Electrophysiol. 2013;24(4):430–6.
28. Kwong RY, et al. Impact of unrecognized myocardial scar detected by cardiac magnetic resonance

imaging on event-free survival in patients presenting with signs or symptoms of coronary artery disease. Circulation. 2006;113(23):2733–43.
29. Klem I, et al. Assessment of myocardial scarring improves risk stratification in patients evaluated for cardiac defibrillator implantation. J Am Coll Cardiol. 2012;60(5):408–20.
30. Salmanipour A, et al. The predictive value of cardiac MRI strain parameters in hypertrophic cardiomyopathy patients with preserved left ventricular ejection fraction and a low fibrosis burden: a retrospective cohort study. Front Cardiovasc Med. 2023:10.
31. Yan AT, et al. Characterization of the peri-infarct zone by contrast-enhanced cardiac magnetic resonance imaging is a powerful predictor of post–myocardial infarction mortality. Circulation. 2006;114(1):32–9.
32. Wu KC, et al. Combined cardiac magnetic resonance imaging and C-reactive protein levels identify a cohort at low risk for defibrillator firings and death. Circ Cardiovasc Imaging. 2012;5(2):178–86.
33. Demirel F, et al. Myocardial scar characteristics based on cardiac magnetic resonance imaging is associated with ventricular tachyarrhythmia in patients with ischemic cardiomyopathy. Int J Cardiol. 2014;177(2):392–9.
34. Antiochos P, et al. Entropy as a measure of myocardial tissue heterogeneity in patients with ventricular arrhythmias. JACC Cardiovasc Imaging. 2022;15(5):783–92.
35. Robbers LF, et al. Myocardial infarct heterogeneity assessment by late gadolinium enhancement cardiovascular magnetic resonance imaging shows predictive value for ventricular arrhythmia development after acute myocardial infarction. Eur Heart J Cardiovasc Imaging. 2013;14(12):1150–8.
36. Taylor AJ, et al. T1 mapping. JACC Cardiovasc Imaging. 2016;9(1):67–81.
37. Middlekauff HR, et al. Syncope in advanced heart failure: high risk of sudden death regardless of origin of syncope. J Am Coll Cardiol. 1993;21(1):110–6.
38. Køber L, et al. Defibrillator implantation in patients with nonischemic systolic heart failure. N Engl J Med. 2016;375(13):1221–30.
39. Kadish A, et al. Prophylactic defibrillator implantation in patients with nonischemic dilated cardiomyopathy. N Engl J Med. 2004;350(21):2151–8.
40. Theerasuwipakorn N, et al. Impact of late gadolinium-enhanced cardiac MRI on arrhythmic and mortality outcomes in nonischemic dilated cardiomyopathy: updated systematic review and meta-analysis. Sci Rep. 2023;13(1):13775.
41. Leyva F, et al. Myocardial fibrosis predicts ventricular arrhythmias and sudden death after cardiac electronic device implantation. J Am Coll Cardiol. 2022;79(7):665–78.
42. Flett A, et al. BRITISH, an ongoing randomised trial of implantable defibrillators for non-ischemic cardiomyopathy with severe LV impairment and myocardial scar: trial design and update. J Cardiovasc Magn Reson. 2025;27
43. Cadour F, et al. Prognostic value of cardiovascular magnetic resonance T1 mapping and extracellular volume fraction in nonischemic dilated cardiomyopathy. J Cardiovasc Magn Reson. 2023;25(1):7.
44. Rubiś PP, et al. Extracellular volume is an independent predictor of arrhythmic burden in dilated cardiomyopathy. Sci Rep. 2021;11(1):24000.
45. Puntmann VO, et al. T1-mapping and outcome in nonischemic cardiomyopathy. JACC Cardiovasc Imaging. 2016;9(1):40–50.
46. Li S, et al. T1 mapping and extracellular volume fraction in dilated cardiomyopathy: a prognosis study. JACC Cardiovasc Imaging. 2022;15(4):578–90.
47. Kiaos A, et al. Prognostic value of cardiovascular magnetic resonance T1 mapping techniques in non-ischemic dilated cardiomyopathy: a systematic review and meta-analysis. Int J Cardiol. 2020;312:110–6.
48. Shen H, et al. Ventricular arrhythmia and sudden cardiac death in hypertrophic cardiomyopathy: from bench to bedside. Front Cardiovasc Med. 2022;9:949294.
49. Segev A, et al. Ventricular arrhythmias in patients with hypertrophic cardiomyopathy: prevalence, distribution, predictors, and outcome. Heart Rhythm. 2023;20(10):1385–92.
50. Falasconi G, et al. Atrial fibrillation in hypertrophic cardiomyopathy: pathophysiology, diagnosis and management. Am J Cardiovasc Dis. 2020;10(4):409–18.
51. Basso C, et al. Arrhythmogenic right ventricular cardiomyopathy. Lancet. 2009;373(9671):1289–300.
52. Oechslin EN, et al. Long-term follow-up of 34 adults with isolated left ventricular noncompaction: a distinct cardiomyopathy with poor prognosis. J Am Coll Cardiol. 2000;36(2):493–500.
53. Towbin JA, Jefferies JL. Cardiomyopathies due to left ventricular noncompaction, mitochondrial and storage diseases, and inborn errors of metabolism. Circ Res. 2017;121(7):838–54.
54. Jolfayi AG, et al. Exploring TTN variants as genetic insights into cardiomyopathy pathogenesis and potential emerging clues to molecular mechanisms in cardiomyopathies. Sci Rep. 2024;14(1):5313.
55. Gersh BJ, et al. 2011 ACCF/AHA guideline for the diagnosis and treatment of hypertrophic cardiomyopathy. Circulation. 2011;124(24):e783–831.
56. Elliott PM, et al. Sudden death in hypertrophic cardiomyopathy: identification of high risk patients. J Am Coll Cardiol. 2000;36(7):2212–8.
57. Pennell DJ. Cardiovascular magnetic resonance. Circulation. 2010;121(5):692–705.
58. Maron BJ. Contemporary insights and strategies for risk stratification and prevention of sudden death in hypertrophic cardiomyopathy. Circulation. 2010;121(3):445–56.

59. Elliott PM, et al. Left ventricular outflow tract obstruction and sudden death risk in patients with hypertrophic cardiomyopathy. Eur Heart J. 2006;27(16):1933–41.
60. Adabag AS, et al. Occurrence and frequency of arrhythmias in hypertrophic cardiomyopathy in relation to delayed enhancement on cardiovascular magnetic resonance. J Am Coll Cardiol. 2008;51(14):1369–74.
61. Chan RH, et al. Prognostic value of quantitative contrast-enhanced cardiovascular magnetic resonance for the evaluation of sudden death risk in patients with hypertrophic cardiomyopathy. Circulation. 2014;130(6):484–95.
62. Weng Z, et al. Prognostic value of LGE-CMR in HCM: a meta-analysis. JACC Cardiovasc Imaging. 2016;9(12):1392–402.
63. Corrado D, Basso C, Judge DP. Arrhythmogenic cardiomyopathy. Circ Res. 2017;121(7):784–802.
64. Aquaro GD, et al. Prognostic value of magnetic resonance phenotype in patients with Arrhythmogenic right ventricular cardiomyopathy. J Am Coll Cardiol. 2020;75(22):2753–65.
65. Corrado D, et al. Diagnosis of arrhythmogenic cardiomyopathy: the Padua criteria. Int J Cardiol. 2020;319:106–14.
66. Mavrogeni SI, et al. The pivotal role of cardiovascular imaging in the identification and risk stratification of non-compaction cardiomyopathy patients. Heart Fail Rev. 2020;25(6):1007–15.
67. Andreini D, et al. Long-term prognostic value of cardiac magnetic resonance in left ventricle noncompaction. J Am Coll Cardiol. 2016;68(20):2166–81.
68. Femia G, et al. Long term clinical outcomes associated with CMR quantified isolated left ventricular non-compaction in adults. Int J Cardiol. 2021;328:235–40.
69. Ramchand J, et al. Novel approach to risk stratification in left ventricular non-compaction using a combined cardiac imaging and plasma biomarker approach. J Am Heart Assoc. 2021;10(8):e019209.
70. Casas G, et al. A comprehensive CMR analysis improves risk stratification in left ventricular noncompaction. Eur Heart J. 2023;44(Suppl 2):ehad655-200.
71. Petersen SE, et al. Excessive Trabeculation of the left ventricle: JACC: cardiovascular imaging expert panel paper. JACC Cardiovasc Imaging. 2023;16(3):408–25.
72. Demirkiran A, et al. Clinical intra-cardiac 4D flow CMR: acquisition, analysis, and clinical applications. Eur Heart J Cardiovasc Imaging. 2021;23(2):154–65.
73. Masoomi Z, et al. Prevalence of contrast-induced nephropathy after primary percutaneous coronary intervention at a tertiary referral hospital. Heliyon. 2024;10(4)
74. Järvensivu-Koivunen M, et al. Ventricular arrhythmias and haemodynamic collapse during acute coronary syndrome: increased risk for sudden cardiac death? Eur J Prev Cardiol. 2024;
75. Al-Khatib SM, et al. 2017 AHA/ACC/HRS guideline for Management of Patients with ventricular arrhythmias and the prevention of sudden cardiac death: a report of the American College of Cardiology/American Heart Association task force on clinical practice guidelines and the Heart Rhythm Society. J Am Coll Cardiol. 2018;72(14):e91–e220.
76. Kunutsor SK, et al. Hemodynamic gain index and risk of ventricular arrhythmias: a prospective cohort study. Scand Cardiovasc J. 2024;58(1):2347289.
77. Holmström L, et al. Artificial intelligence in ventricular arrhythmias and sudden death. Arrhythm Electrophysiol Rev. 2023;12:e17.
78. Cha Y-M, et al. Machine learning for prediction of ventricular arrhythmia episodes from intracardiac electrograms of automatic implantable cardioverter-defibrillators. Heart Rhythm. 2024;
79. Mohanty M, Biswal P, Sabut S. Machine learning approach to recognize ventricular arrhythmias using VMD based features. Multidim Syst Sign Process. 2020;31(1):49–71.
80. Li L, et al. Use of machine learning algorithms to predict life-threatening ventricular arrhythmia in sepsis. Eur Heart J Digit Health. 2023;4(3):245–53.
81. Montalt-Tordera J, et al. Machine learning in magnetic resonance imaging: image reconstruction. Phys Med. 2021;83:79–87.
82. Popescu DM, et al. Arrhythmic sudden death survival prediction using deep learning analysis of scarring in the heart. Nat Cardiovasc Res. 2022;1(4):334–43.
83. Pfeffer A, et al. Machine learning score using cardiac MRI to predict cardiovascular events in patients with acute myocarditis. Arch Cardiovasc Dis. 2024;117(Suppl 1):S56.
84. O'Mahony C, et al. A novel clinical risk prediction model for sudden cardiac death in hypertrophic cardiomyopathy (HCM risk-SCD). Eur Heart J. 2014;35(30):2010–20.
85. Alis D, et al. Assessment of ventricular tachyarrhythmia in patients with hypertrophic cardiomyopathy with machine learning-based texture analysis of late gadolinium enhancement cardiac MRI. Diagn Interv Imaging. 2020;101(3):137–46.
86. Khurshid S, et al. Deep learning to predict cardiac magnetic resonance–derived left ventricular mass and hypertrophy from 12-lead ECGs. Circ Cardiovasc Imaging. 2021;14(6):e012281.
87. Akyea RK, et al. Arrhythmic mitral valve prolapse phenotype: an unsupervised machine learning analysis using a multicenter cardiac MRI registry. Radiol Cardiothoracic Imaging. 2024;6(3):e230247.
88. Kolk MZH, et al. Multimodal explainable artificial intelligence identifies patients with non-ischaemic cardiomyopathy at risk of lethal ventricular arrhythmias. Sci Rep. 2024;14(1):14889.
89. Van Lieshout FE, et al. Deep learning for ventricular arrhythmia prediction using fibrosis segmentations on cardiac MRI data. In: 2022 computing in cardiology (CinC). IEEE; 2022.

90. Krebs J, et al. CinE caRdiac magneTic resonAnce to predIct veNTricular arrhYthmia (CERTAINTY). Sci Rep. 2021;11(1):22683.
91. Pirruccello JP, et al. Deep learning of left atrial structure and function provides link to atrial fibrillation risk. Nat Commun. 2024;15(1):4304.
92. Raman SV, et al. Volumetric cine CMR to quantify atrial structure and function in patients with atrial dysrhythmias. J Cardiovasc Magn Reson. 2005;7(3):539–43.
93. Nakao R, et al. Relation of left atrial flow, volume, and strain to paroxysmal atrial fibrillation in patients with hypertrophic cardiomyopathy. Am J Cardiol. 2022;166:72–80.
94. Laubrock K, et al. Imaging of arrhythmia: real-time cardiac magnetic resonance imaging in atrial fibrillation. Eur J Radiol Open. 2022;9:100404.
95. DiCarlo AL, et al. Assessment of beat-to-beat variability in left atrial hemodynamics using real time phase contrast MRI in patients with atrial fibrillation. J Magn Reson Imaging. 2023;58(3):763–71.
96. Guensch DP, et al. Analysis of bi-atrial function using CMR feature tracking and long-axis shortening approaches in patients with diastolic dysfunction and atrial fibrillation. Eur Radiol. 2023;33(10):7226–37.
97. Mojica-Pisciotti ML, et al. Left atrium phasic impairments in paroxysmal atrial fibrillation patients assessed by cardiovascular magnetic resonance feature tracking. Sci Rep. 2022;12(1):7539.
98. Habibi M, et al. CMR-measured left atrial volume and function and incident atrial fibrillation: results from the multi-ethnic study of atherosclerosis (MESA). Circ Cardiovasc Imaging. 2016;9(8)
99. Caixal G, et al. Accuracy of left atrial fibrosis detection with cardiac magnetic resonance: correlation of late gadolinium enhancement with endocardial voltage and conduction velocity. Europace. 2021;23(3):380–8.
100. Letsas K, et al. Cardiovascular magnetic resonance 3D LGE imaging for atrial fibrillation ablation. Europace. 2024;26(Suppl 1):euae102. 201.
101. Nyktari E, et al. Cardiovascular magnetic resonance 3D LGE imaging for atrial fibrillation ablation understanding left atrial structural changes. J Cardiovasc Magn Reson. 2024;26
102. Charafeddine F, Refaat MM. Cardiac magnetic resonance T1 mapping for prediction of atrial fibrillation recurrence after cryoablation. Pacing Clin Electrophysiol. 2020;43(2):167–8.
103. Spartera M, et al. Left atrial 4D flow cardiovascular magnetic resonance: a reproducibility study in sinus rhythm and atrial fibrillation. J Cardiovasc Magn Reson. 2021;23(1):29.
104. Markl M, et al. Left atrial and left atrial appendage 4D blood flow dynamics in atrial fibrillation. Circ Cardiovasc Imaging. 2016;9(9):e004984.
105. Demirkiran A, et al. Altered left atrial 4D flow characteristics in patients with paroxysmal atrial fibrillation in the absence of apparent remodeling. Sci Rep. 2021;11(1):5965.
106. Dohy Z, et al. Feasibility and image quality of bright-blood and black-blood phase-sensitive inversion recovery (BOOST) sequence in clinical practice using for left atrial visualization in patients with atrial fibrillation. Eur Radiol. 2024;34(4):2689–98.
107. Ghaffari Jolfayi A, et al. Imaging findings in cardiovascular involvements of IgG4-related disease: a systematic review study. Rheumatology. 2024;
108. Chalian H, et al. The role of cardiac magnetic resonance imaging parameters in prognostication of systemic sclerosis in patients with cardiac involvement: a systematic review of the literature. Acad Radiol. 2024;
109. Deux J-F, et al. Simultaneous bright-and black-blood whole-heart (BOOST) MRI to demarcate left atrial ablated tissue immediately after RadioFBequency catheter ablation without administered intravenous contrast media. J Cardiovasc Magn Reson. 2024;26
110. Pezel T, et al. Feasibility and prognostic value of vasodilator stress perfusion CMR in patients with atrial fibrillation. Cardiovasc Imaging. 2021;14(2):379–89.
111. Nelsson A, et al. Pulmonary blood volume measured by cardiovascular magnetic resonance: influence of pulmonary transit time methods and left atrial volume. J Cardiovasc Magn Reson. 2021;23(1):123.
112. Dykstra S, et al. Machine learning prediction of atrial fibrillation in cardiovascular patients using cardiac magnetic resonance and electronic health information. Front Cardiovasc Med. 2022;9:998558.
113. Pujadas ER, et al. Prediction of incident cardiovascular events using machine learning and CMR radiomics. Eur Radiol. 2023;33(5):3488–500.
114. Miao F, et al. Is random survival Forest an alternative to cox proportional model on predicting cardiovascular disease? In: 6th European conference of the International Federation for Medical and Biological Engineering. Cham: Springer; 2015.
115. Fan X, et al. Predictive value of machine learning for recurrence of atrial fibrillation after catheter ablation: a systematic review and meta-analysis. Rev Cardiovasc Med. 2023;24(11):315.
116. Elahi R, Nazari M. An updated overview of radiomics-based artificial intelligence (AI) methods in breast cancer screening and diagnosis. Radiol Phys Technol. 2024;17(4):795–818.
117. Valizadeh G, et al. Deep learning approaches for early prediction of conversion from MCI to AD using MRI and clinical data: a systematic review. Arch Comput Methods Eng. 2024;
118. Pujadas ER, et al. Atrial fibrillation prediction by combining ECG markers and CMR radiomics. Sci Rep. 2022;12(1):18876.
119. Jing M, et al. Value of imaging in the non-invasive prediction of recurrence after catheter ablation in patients with atrial fibrillation: an up-to-date review. Rev Cardiovasc Med. 2023;24(8):241.

6 The Role of AI and Cardiac Magnetic Resonance Imaging in Identifying Inflammatory Heart Disease

Amir Ghaffari Jolfayi, Hamed Ghoshouni, Mahshad Sarikhani, Ali Jafari, Alireza Salmanipour, and Golnaz Houshmand

Abstract

The integration of Artificial Intelligence (AI) and advanced imaging technologies is reshaping the landscape of cardiovascular medicine, offering transformative approaches to the diagnosis, management, and prognosis of complex cardiac conditions. The convergence of AI and cardiac magnetic resonance (CMR) imaging has enhanced diagnostic precision, automated image analysis, and personalized treatment strategies for inflammatory cardiovascular diseases like myocarditis, pericarditis, and autoimmune rheumatologic conditions with cardiac involvement conditions like sarcoidosis, and systemic lupus erythematosus (SLE).

AI-driven methodologies, particularly machine learning (ML) and deep learning (DL) algorithms, have demonstrated remarkable efficacy in identifying subtle pathological changes, detecting and quantifying myocardial inflammation, and predicting disease outcomes with unprecedented accuracy. Innovations such as convolutional neural networks (CNNs) and hybrid models like CNN-KCL significantly enhance CMR's capabilities, enabling early detection and reducing diagnostic variability. By analyzing complex imaging datasets, AI supports comprehensive tissue characterization, advancing the understanding of inflammatory processes and myocardial remodeling.

The article also explores AI's potential in risk stratification and outcome prediction, emphasizing its role in aligning with personalized medicine principles. Despite the promise, challenges such as dataset limitations, model explainability, and the need for multicenter validation persist, underscoring the importance of collaborative efforts in AI development.

Keywords

Cardiac magnetic resonance imaging · Inflammatory heart disease · Deep learning · Machine learning · Artificial intelligence · Fibrosis · Myocarditis · Pericarditis · Systemic lupus erythrocytosis · Sarcoidosis

Authors Amir Ghaffari Jolfayi, Hamed Ghoshouni have contributed equality and shared the first co-authorship.

A. Ghaffari Jolfayi · H. Ghoshouni · A. Salmanipour
G. Houshmand (✉)
Cardiovascular Imaging Research Center, Rajaie Cardiovascular Institute, Tehran, Iran

M. Sarikhani
Department of Radiology, Shariati Hospital, Tehran University of Medical Sciences, Tehran, Iran

A. Jafari
School of Medicine, Shahid Beheshti University of Medical Sciences, Tehran, Iran

A. Ghaffari Jolfayi (ed.), *Navigating Cardiology's Future*,
https://doi.org/10.1007/978-981-95-0313-1_6

6.1 Introduction

Inflammatory heart diseases encompass a range of conditions that affect the heart's tissues due to inflammation, often triggered by infections, autoimmune responses, or other systemic disorders [1]. Myocarditis involves inflammation of the heart muscle (myocardium), often caused by viral infections, autoimmune diseases, or toxins, and can lead to heart failure, arrhythmias, or sudden death in severe cases [2]. Pericarditis refers to inflammation of the pericardium, the sac surrounding the heart, and is characterized by sharp chest pain that worsens with breathing or lying down, often caused by infections, autoimmune conditions, or trauma [3]. Sarcoidosis, a multi-system inflammatory disease, can involve the heart, leading to granulomas (clusters of immune cells) in the myocardium, potentially causing arrhythmias, heart block, or heart failure [4]. Systemic Lupus Erythematosus (SLE), a chronic autoimmune disease, frequently affects the heart, contributing to conditions such as pericarditis, myocarditis, or valvular dysfunction due to immune-mediated damage. These diseases require timely diagnosis and management to mitigate complications and preserve cardiac function [5].

Cardiovascular magnetic resonance (CMR) is a potent imaging tool to assess the cardiac structure and heart function in various heart conditions, including inflammatory heart disease. Different AI methods focus on various aspects of the imaging process, such as segmentation, reconstruction, motion, and deformation analysis. On the other hand, other AI projects concentrate on providing faster and more accurate diagnoses. These projects facilitate deep-learning/machine-learning structures such as the Convolutional Neural Network (CNN). CNN mimics neural connectivity patterns in the visual cortex of the human brain. As it is comprehensible, CNNs are used for computer vision, image recognition, object detection, and medical image analysis. A convolutional layer is the foundation of CNN in which image processing occurs for each image property (edges, textures, or colors). For each property, a specific convolutional layer may be needed. Deeper layers receive processed data from the previous layers, thus recognizing more complex properties such as patterns and movements [6].

Inflammatory heart diseases represent complex conditions that demand accurate diagnosis and targeted management to prevent adverse outcomes. Advances in imaging technologies, particularly cardiovascular magnetic resonance (CMR) and positron Emission Tomography (PET), have revolutionized the evaluation of cardiac inflammation, enabling detailed insights into heart function and structure. The integration of Artificial Intelligence (AI), especially through techniques like convolutional neural networks (CNNs), has further enhanced diagnostic precision by automating image analysis and recognizing intricate patterns of inflammation and dysfunction. These innovations hold promise for improving patient outcomes by facilitating early intervention, personalized treatment, and better monitoring of inflammatory heart diseases.

6.2 AI in Quantifying Inflammation: From Edema and Fibrosis Towards the Management

Inflammatory heart diseases present significant diagnostic challenges due to their complex and often confusing clinical manifestations. Accurate detection and quantification of inflammation are crucial for timely intervention and effective management, as these conditions can lead to severe complications such as heart failure and sudden cardiac death if left untreated. Traditionally, the diagnosis of inflammation has relied on invasive procedures like endomyocardial biopsies (EMB) and remains the gold standard, as it provides tissue diagnosis. CMR provides a valuable tool for detecting inflammation through techniques like parametric mapping and late gadolinium imaging and advanced techniques, and provides a non-invasive method for tissue characterization and detecting inflammation and fibrosis. However, these methods have limitations, including limited sensitivity, and potential for subjective interpretation. Recent advancements in AI have significantly enhanced the capabilities of CMR, offering a transformative approach to diagnosing and quantifying inflammation in cardiac diseases. By integrating machine learning (ML) and deep learning (DL) algorithms with CMR, clinicians can achieve advanced tissue characterization, enabling the detection of inflammatory processes like myocardial edema and fibrosis with unprecedented accuracy [7, 8].

AI algorithms, particularly those based on ML and DL, can process vast amounts of imaging data to detect patterns and anomalies imperceptible to humans. Notably, AI-driven tools aid in the analysis of complex imaging datasets, extracting valuable diagnostic and prognostic information that surpasses traditional imaging techniques in speed and accuracy. For example, the CNN-KCL model, which combines CNN with k-means clustering (KCL), has significantly improved myocarditis diagnosis, achieving an accuracy rate of more than 90%. This model effectively segments and analyzes imaging data, emphasizing its potential to handle complex clinical data efficiently [8, 9].

Sharifrazi et al. considered CMR the gold standard non-invasive diagnostic tool for myocarditis, aiming to improve this technique through Computer-aided diagnosis (CAD). Their study studied 98,898 images taken from 47 subjects utilizing a CNN module that resulted in 97.41% accuracy in the diagnosis of myocarditis. That means CAD performed with a higher accuracy rate than human cardiac imaging experts. The study employed a K-means clustering approach with varying clusters to optimize the diagnostic performance of a CNN. The 2-cluster method (healthy vs. afflicted) demonstrated low accuracy, while increasing clusters improved diagnostic precision. The CNN consisted of 12 layers, including 3 convolutional layers, 3 max-pooling layers, and 4 dropout layers to mitigate overfitting. This configuration achieved a high diagnostic reliability of 97.41% [10].

In a different machine learning approach, Moravvej et al. facilitated an artificial bee colony algorithm (ABC) and performed reinforcement learning instead of the standard deep learning approach. For this study, the diagnosis of myocarditis on CMR was based on Lake Louise criteria. By employing ABC, they created three individual CNNs as Bees in their colony and then a feed-forward network with three hidden layers. As the ABC algorithm is defined, the feed-forward network has to choose the best solution created by the three CNNs. Also, the total number of patients in this study was 586, and they have entered 307 healthy candidates as controls. All of the CMR images in this study were resized to 100*100 for input normalization [11].

6.2.1 T1 and T2 Mapping

In CMR, AI algorithms analyze quantitative imaging parameters such as T1 and T2 relaxation times, which are altered by inflammatory processes in the myocardium. In myocarditis, AI-driven CMR can quantify the degree of myocardial damage and inflammation by assessing myocardial edema and hyperemia using T1 and T2 mapping techniques. Incorporating novel multiparametric imaging approaches, such as combining T2 mapping with CMR feature tracking, has been shown to increase diagnostic sensitivity in acute myocarditis compared to traditional methods. These approaches leverage the strengths of different imaging modalities to provide a more comprehensive assessment of myocardial inflammation, potentially outperforming conventional Lake Louise Criteria by integrating T2 mapping-derived parameters like mean absolute deviation (MAD) of segmental pixel-SD (madSD) with strain parameters like global circumferential strain (GCS) of the left ventricle and LGE. Such multiparametric methods exemplify the significant role of AI in enhancing the precision of CMR, paving the way for more personalized and effective treatment strategies [12].

6.2.2 Fibrosis and LGE

Deep learning algorithms excel in analyzing LGE images, which are commonly used in CMR to detect areas of myocardial fibrosis [13]. These areas of fibrosis, which result from myocardial inflammation, can be visualized due to the retention of gadolinium contrast agents in damaged myocardium. Through pattern recognition, AI models can differentiate between healthy and pathological myocardial tissue with a high degree of accuracy. This is especially important in diseases like cardiac sarcoidosis, where inflammation may present in a heterogeneous and patchy distribution across the myocardium, making it challenging for endomyocardial biopsy or noninvasive parametric mapping to provide a clear assessment. AI algorithms enhance this process by identifying the extent and distribution of myocardial involvement more reliably than human observers alone [9, 12].

6.2.3 Personalized Medicine in Monitoring Progression and Response to Treatment

The application of AI-driven CMR extends beyond diagnosis and significantly impacts patient management. AI-driven models can predict disease progression and response to therapy by quantifying subtle changes in myocardial tissue character and function. This capability is crucial for conditions like sarcoidosis and myocarditis, where inflammation can lead to significant cardiac dysfunction or life-threatening arrhythmia over time. AI-enhanced imaging can monitor disease progression and response to treatment by tracking changes in myocardial inflammation over time in diseases like cardiac sarcoidosis. Thus, AI supports a more tailored approach to patient care, aligning with the broader goals of personalized medicine. Moreover, AI algorithms reduce the subjectivity associated with human interpretation by automating aspects of image analysis. This automation increases diagnostic throughput and minimizes inter-observer variability, leading to more consistent and reliable results for tracking disease progression and evaluating therapeutic efficacy over time. By overcoming limitations of human interpretation, such as variability and potential for error, AI makes the diagnostic and monitoring process more precise and reliable [9, 14, 15].

6.2.4 AI in Predicting Long-Term Outcomes and Personalized Treatment in Pericardial Inflammation

AI has significant potential in predicting the progression of pericarditis to chronic forms, such as constrictive pericarditis. By analyzing CMR data along with serial clinical markers, AI models can predict which patients are at higher risk of developing constrictive pericarditis and may benefit from earlier intervention. Additionally, AI-driven models can help personalize treatment strategies by predicting patient responses to colchicine or steroids, allowing for more tailored therapeutic regimens [16, 17]. This is particularly valuable in cases of recurrent pericarditis, where prolonged treatment may be necessary to prevent relapses.

6.3 Prognostic Value and Outcome Prediction of AI-Driven CMR in Inflammatory Heart Disease

The ability of AI to process and interpret massive datasets, including imaging, clinical, and biochemical data, offers a novel approach to both diagnosis and prognosis in inflammatory heart disease [15]. These tools can learn from vast amounts of data, identify patterns, and make predictions that can improve diagnostic accuracy and prognostic stratification. Furthermore, AI models can integrate imaging data with other clinical parameters (e.g., biomarker levels, genetic information, and patient demographics), providing a more comprehensive view of the patient's condition and enabling personalized treatment strategies [16, 17]. Adopting Explainable AI (XAI) techniques, such as Gradient-weighted Class Activation Mapping (Grad-CAM), is essential to enhance the transparency of AI models and foster clinician trust in AI-assisted decision-making [18, 19].

6.3.1 AI-Driven CMR Models in Myocarditis

Myocarditis is a condition in which the middle layer of the heart wall, the myocardium, is inflamed, and viral infections are considered the main culprits in this process. This inflammation can alter the electrical system in the myocardium and its synchronous function [2, 20]. Despite all progress in cardiology, myocarditis has remained one of the most challenging cardiology diagnoses. The clinical manifestations of myocarditis, which are chest pain and mild dyspnea, are common among cardiovascular diseases. CMR is the gold standard imaging tool for myocarditis diagnosis because of its non-invasive nature and the superb data it can provide about myocardial mechanical and functional disturbances [21].

Early Diagnosis Myocarditis is one of the most widely studied inflammatory heart diseases, with clinical manifestations ranging from asymptomatic disease to fulminant cardiac failure, arrhythmias, or sudden cardiac death [22]. Traditionally, endomyocardial biopsy (EMB) has been regarded as the gold standard for diagnosing myocarditis, but its invasive nature and associated risks, such as false positives, false negatives, and sampling errors, limit its widespread use. As a result, non-invasive techniques like CMR are increasingly being adopted for diagnosis [23]. CMR offers valuable insights through imaging markers such as LGE, T1 and T2 mapping, and global longitudinal strain (GLS) [23–25]. However, traditional CMR interpretation is heavily reliant on expert radiologists/cardiologists, and interobserver variability is a significant drawback [26].

It is crucial to detect cardiac diseases as soon as possible, as the earlier the diagnosis, the lower the mortality rate [27]. Clinics' technical limitations and clinicians' heavy workloads may lead to invisible lesions or misdiagnosis [28]. Machine Learning techniques can help us improve the accuracy of myocarditis diagnosis. This approach, also called computer-aided diagnosis, aims to accelerate the diagnosis of this medical condition.

Myocarditis Identification in CMR To describe the myocarditis, we use the Lake Louise Criteria (LLC), which is based on three findings in CMR: myocardial edema, hyperemia/capillary leak, and scar. Each specific diagnostic target is shown in one of the MRI images. Myocardial injury can be seen with late gadolinium enhancement (LGE); on the other hand, T2-weighted images can affirm interstitial edema, and T1-weighted images can indicate hyperemia/capillary leak [29].

The JACC Scientific Expert Panel has updated the CMR diagnostic criteria for detecting myocardial inflammation in patients with suspected acute or active myocardial inflammation (Lake Louise Criteria). The new recommendations include parametric mapping techniques and emphasize that combining CMR markers improves diagnostic specificity. Specifically, evidence of myocardial inflammation is more substantial if both a T2-based marker (e.g., increased T2 relaxation time or signal intensity) and a T1-based marker (e.g., elevated T1, extracellular volume, or late gadolinium enhancement) are present. While having both markers provides higher specificity, a single marker may still support a diagnosis in appropriate clinical contexts, though with less specificity. These updates aim to enhance the accuracy of CMR in diagnosing myocardial inflammation [29–31].

6.3.1.1 Diagnostic Applications of AI in Myocarditis

AI, particularly DL and ML techniques, can overcome these limitations by enhancing diagnostic accuracy, reducing diagnostic time, and minimizing inter-observer variability [23, 32]. Several AI models have been employed in diagnostic studies, most notably CNNs, Generative Adversarial Networks (GANs), and Reinforcement Learning algorithms [33]. CNNs are particularly effective in analyzing medical images, enabling the detection of myocarditis with high sensitivity and specificity. GANs have also been employed to improve the quality of CMR images, making the diagnosis more reliable. In addition, Support Vector Machines (SVMs) and Random Forests (RFs) have been used to analyze ECG data and other clinical variables, achieving high diagnostic performance [23, 34–36].

LGE, a hallmark of myocardial fibrosis, is a well-established imaging marker in myocarditis and a predictor of adverse outcomes [25]. AI models can automate the detection and quantification of LGE, reducing observer variability and improving reproducibility. Additionally, AI can assist in refining T1 and T2 mapping, which are sensitive to myocardial edema and fibrosis, by automating the interpretation of myocardial relaxation times and enabling more accurate differentiation between acute and chronic myocarditis [37, 38]. Moreover, AI can enhance the extraction of global longitudinal strain (GLS), an early marker of myocardial dysfunction, by automating the measurement of myocardial deformation [39]. This allows for earlier detection of subtle changes in myocardial function that may not yet be detectable with traditional markers.

The key findings from the reviewed studies indicate that AI models can achieve diagnostic accuracy rates of up to 90% in distinguishing myocarditis from other conditions, such as myocardial infarction [40]. AI-enhanced CMR analysis has significantly reduced the diagnosis time, which is especially critical in acute cases of myocarditis, where rapid intervention can be lifesaving. Moreover, AI models have been shown to reduce inter-observer variability, making the diagnostic process more consistent and reliable [23].

Early detection of myocarditis is the key to reducing the risk of developing dilated cardiomyopathy or chronic active inflammation of the myocardium. The only precise diagnostic tool for proving the existence of myocarditis is an endomyocardial biopsy, which is decisive but invasive at the same time [41].

In a 2018 study by Baessler et al., CMR was compared to traditional endomyocardial biopsy in diagnosing acute myocarditis among 39 patients. While endomyocardial biopsy confirmed myocarditis in 26 cases, the diagnostic performance of CMR metrics such as T1, T2, and LGE was relatively low, with AUC values ranging from 0.62 to 0.67 for T2 and T1 mapping, respectively. However, combining CMR texture features, specifically T2 run-length non-uniformity and gray-level non-uniformity, significantly improved diagnostic accuracy, achieving an AUC of 0.88, sensitivity of 89%, and specificity of 92% [41].

Despite these advancements, several challenges remained to be dealt with. Variability in CMR scan quality—due to differences in imaging protocols, image sizes, and parameters—can influence the performance of AI models. Additionally, most studies rely on data from single-center cohorts, which limits the generalizability of the findings. There is a need for multicenter datasets to ensure that AI models are robust and can be applied to a broader population.

6.3.1.2 Risk Stratification and Predicting Adverse Outcomes

AI models have also shown potential in predicting survival outcomes in myocarditis patients, particularly in high-risk populations such as pediatric cases or emergency settings [42, 43]. In this context, AI-based models have been employed to predict major adverse cardiac events (MACE) and the need for prompt interventions [42, 44]. Popular AI models for survival prediction include RF and Deep Neural Networks (DNNs), which can analyze large datasets with multiple variables to assess patient risk. For example, in a study on pediatric populations, Random Forest models demonstrated AUC values exceeding 0.9 when predicting survival outcomes [43].

The strength of AI lies in its ability to integrate disparate data sources into predictive models. AI-driven algorithms can stratify patients with myocarditis according to their risk of developing complications, such as heart failure, ventricular arrhythmias, or sudden cardiac death [45, 46]. For instance, AI can analyze the extent of LGE, combined with clinical and biochemical data, to predict which patients are at higher risk of progressing to dilated cardiomyopathy or experiencing life-threatening arrhythmias [23]. Additionally, AI can aid in predicting the transition from acute to chronic myocarditis by identifying persistent inflammation or fibrosis even when clinical symptoms have resolved, informing decisions on the need for immunosuppressive therapy or implantable cardioverter-defibrillators (ICDs) [23].

6.3.2 AI-Driven CMR Models in Pericarditis

Pericarditis is an inflammatory condition affecting the pericardium, which can present acutely or evolve into chronic forms such as constrictive pericarditis [47]. Accurately diagnosing and managing pericarditis relies heavily on CMR, which can detect pericardial thickening, effusion, and inflammation—all key indicators of disease severity [48]. However, as with other IHDs, CMR interpretation in pericarditis can be challenging, and AI offers the potential to enhance diagnostic accuracy and prognostic assessments.

6.3.2.1 Enhanced Detection of Pericardial Inflammation and Effusion

AI-driven models can automate the identification of pericardial thickening and effusion, improving the sensitivity of CMR in detecting pericardial inflammation. This is particularly important in cases where pericardial involvement is subtle or where there is a need to differentiate between pericarditis and pericardial effusion secondary to other causes, such as heart failure or renal failure [49]. There are limited studies on CMR for the detection of pericarditis, and instead, studies are mostly focused on ECG.

For instance, Liu et al. developed a DLM to detect acute pericarditis using 12-lead electrocardiograms and compared it to human experts and traditional machine learning models. The DLM, trained on raw ECG signals, outperformed both the Xtreme Gradient Boosting (XGB) model based on traditional ECG features and the Philips automatic ECG algorithm. In the validation set, the DLM achieved an area under the AUC of 0.95, with a sensitivity of 78.9% and specificity of 97.7%. To further improve diagnostic accuracy, the researchers integrated the DLM with a previously developed STEMI-DLM, increasing specificity to 99.4%, demonstrating the effectiveness of AI in distinguishing acute pericarditis from similar cardiac conditions [50].

Moreover, Sengupta et al. conducted a pilot study to evaluate the efficacy of a cognitive machine-learning algorithm in differentiating between constrictive pericarditis and restrictive cardiomyopathy (RCM) using echocardiographic data, including speckle tracking echocardiography (STE). The authors developed an associative memory classifier (AMC) that was trained on multidimensional clinical and echocardiographic variables from 94 patients (50 with CP, 44 with RCM). The AMC algorithm normalized and binned STE data into quintiles and used a multistep process to identify key predictive variables. The classifier achieved an AUC of 89.2% using only STE variables, which increased to 96.2% with the addition of four conventional echocardiographic variables. The AMC demonstrated superior diagnostic accuracy and a shorter learning curve compared to other machine-learning models, such as Random Forest and Support Vector Machines, achieving 90% classification accuracy with just 30 training trials [49].

6.3.3 AI-Driven MRI Models in Sarcoidosis and Autoimmune Heart Diseases

Sarcoidosis and systemic lupus erythematosus (SLE) are systemic inflammatory diseases that frequently involve the heart, leading to myocardial inflammation, fibrosis, and arrhythmias [51]. CMR is a crucial tool for detecting cardiac involvement in these diseases, with LGE serving as a key marker of myocardial fibrosis and inflammation [52]. However, AI can enhance the diagnostic and prognostic capabilities of CMR in these complex scenarios.

6.3.3.1 AI'S Role in Detecting Cardiac Sarcoidosis and Lupus-Related Myocardial Inflammation

AI-driven models can enhance the detection of cardiac sarcoidosis and lupus-related myocardial inflammation by automating the interpretation of LGE and T2 mapping scans [14]. This is particularly important in cases where the cardiac involvement is subclinical, as early detection enables prompt initiation of immunosuppressive therapy, which can prevent further myocardial damage.

A recent review paper provides an overview of the role of CMR imaging in detecting myocardial involvement in SLE. Due to varied clinical presentations, diagnosing SLE-related myocardial conditions, such as lupus myocarditis and subclinical myocardial involvement, is challenging. Traditional diagnostic methods like electrocardiograms and echocardiography have limitations, while endomyocardial biopsy is invasive. CMR offers a non-invasive alternative, effectively identifying myocardial inflammation, fibrosis, and edema using techniques like T1/T2 mapping and LGE [53]. However, despite the promise of CMR in SLE, AI-based CMR applications are still lacking, and further research is needed to explore their potential and standardize their use in clinical settings for SLE-related cardiac conditions.

Regarding sarcoidosis, Eckstein et al. (2023) explored using ML to enhance the diagnosis of cardiac sarcoidosis using CMR-derived multichamber volumetric and strain analyses. The study analyzed data from 107 subjects: 45 CMR-negative sarcoidosis patients, 18 CMR-positive sarcoidosis patients, and 44 healthy controls. Several ML classifiers, including support vector machine, random forest, logistic regression, K-nearest neighbor, decision tree, gradient boosting, extreme gradient boosting (XGBoost), and a Voting classifier, were applied to predict CS based on CMR features. The RF and Voting classifiers demonstrated the highest accuracy (81.82%) in distinguishing between controls, CMR(+), and CMR(−) patients. In a two-group analysis (controls vs. all sarcoidosis patients), logistic regression, RF, and SVM yielded a high accuracy of 96%. However, the distinction between CMR(+) and CMR(−) patients was more challenging, with an initial accuracy of 68%, which improved to 89% with feature selection using logistic regression. The study concluded that ML models, particularly with feature selection, significantly enhance the non-invasive diagnosis of cardiac sarcoidosis, suggesting a higher prevalence of cardiac involvement than previously recognized [14].

6.3.3.2 Risk Stratification and Outcome Prediction in Sarcoidosis and SLE

AI-driven CMR can predict long-term outcomes in patients with cardiac sarcoidosis or SLE by analyzing the extent of fibrosis and inflammation. This is critical for identifying patients at higher risk of developing heart failure or ventricular arrhythmias, which may necessitate more aggressive interventions, such as ICD implantation or immunosuppressive therapy [54].

For instance, based on CMR imaging data, Lu et al. used deep learning and machine learning to predict adverse cardiac events in patients with cardiac sarcoidosis. The study retrospectively analyzed a cohort of 117 sarcoidosis patients, using a deep convolutional neural network (DCNN) for automated image processing to extract 232 LV structural and functional features. Three ML algorithms—logistic regression, support vector machine, and multi-layer neural networks (MLP)—were employed to classify patients based on the risk of adverse events. Automated image processing consistently demonstrated higher predictive accuracy than manual methods, with SVM, LR, and MLP models showing better performance when trained on features derived from automated segmentation [55].

Furthermore, Shade et al. developed the Computational Heart and Artificial Intelligence (CHAI) risk predictor to improve sudden cardiac death risk assessment in patients with cardiac sarcoidosis. Current risk prediction methods, such as LVEF and imaging, often fail to accurately identify high-risk patients, leading to inappropriate use of ICDs. The CHAI Risk Predictor combines personalized 3D heart models from MRI and PET scans with ML. The heart models simulate arrhythmia risk based on fibrosis and inflammation patterns, and an ML classifier integrates these simulations with clinical and imaging data. The ML model, using a random forest algorithm, selects key predictive features, optimizing risk prediction. In a study of 45 patients, the CHAI Predictor achieved 60% sensitivity, 72% specificity, and an AUC of 0.754, outperforming conventional clinical metrics. This approach shows promise for improving SCD risk stratification with AI and reducing unnecessary ICD interventions in CS patients [56].

6.4 Challenges and Future Directions

Despite its promise, AI-driven CMR faces several challenges that must be addressed to ensure its widespread clinical adoption. One of the most significant challenges is the lack of large, multicenter datasets that are necessary to train and validate AI models. Most current models are developed using small, single-center datasets, which limits their generalizability and clinical applicability. Collaborative efforts to establish large, diverse datasets will be essential for developing robust, generalizable AI models.

Another major challenge is the black-box nature of many AI algorithms, making it difficult for clinicians to trust AI-driven predictions. The integration of Explainable AI (XAI) techniques, such as Gradient-weighted Class Activation Mapping (Grad-CAM), can help address this issue by providing visual explanations of how AI models arrive at their predictions. This transparency is crucial for fostering clinician trust and ensuring that AI models are used appropriately in clinical practice.

In addition, inflammatory heart conditions are not very common. Thus, during data training, class imbalance often arises, which can overestimate a model's accuracy compared to real-world models [57–59].

For future studies, investigating a larger number of patients and using other machine-learning methods can change the outcome of the studies, so it is highly recommended that the data source be enlarged for future studies. Some new neural network structures are used for image processing in daily products that are faster and more efficient in processing images than the older CNN methods. It can also be a great opportunity to try these new AI pioneer modules as the main approach for studies.

6.5 Conclusion

The integration of AI into CMR for the diagnosis and prognosis of inflammatory heart diseases represents a transformative development in cardiovascular medicine. AI-driven models can enhance diagnostic accuracy, automate complex image analyses, and provide personalized prognostic insights that guide clinical decision-making. This chapter should provide a comprehensive exploration of how AI can improve the management of inflammatory heart diseases with a focus on the potential for AI to enhance patient outcomes. Future research should prioritize the development of large, multicenter datasets and the integration of Explainable AI tools to ensure that AI-driven models are both reliable and transparent, thereby improving clinical outcomes in patients with inflammatory heart diseases.

References

1. Lu L, Sun R, Liu M, Zheng Y, Zhang P. The inflammatory heart diseases: causes, symptoms, and treatments. Cell Biochem Biophys. 2015;72(3):851–5.
2. Sagar S, Liu PP, Cooper LT Jr. Myocarditis. Lancet. 2012;379(9817):738–47.
3. Dababneh E, Siddique MS. Pericarditis.StatPearls. Treasure Island (FL): StatPearls Publishing. Copyright © 2024, StatPearls Publishing LLC; 2024.
4. Cheng RK, Kittleson MM, Beavers CJ, Birnie DH, Blankstein R, Bravo PE, et al. Diagnosis and management of cardiac sarcoidosis: a scientific statement from the American Heart Association. Circulation. 2024;149(21):e1197–e216.
5. Zagelbaum Ward NK, Linares-Koloffon C, Posligua A, Gandrabur L, Kim WY, Sperber K, et al. Cardiac manifestations of systemic lupus erythematous: an overview of the incidence, risk factors, diagnostic cri-

teria, pathophysiology and treatment options. Cardiol Rev. 2022;30(1):38–43.
6. Mzoughi H, Njeh I, Wali A, Slima MB, BenHamida A, Mhiri C, et al. Deep multi-scale 3D convolutional neural network (CNN) for MRI gliomas brain tumor classification. J Digit Imaging. 2020;33(4):903–15.
7. O'Connor MJ. Imaging the itis: endocarditis, myocarditis, and pericarditis. Curr Opin Cardiol. 2019;34(1):57–64.
8. García Sebastián C, Hinojar Baydés R, Zamorano Gómez JL, Fernández-Golfín LC. Cardiac magnetic resonance for myocardial inflammation: current state and future directions. Curr Cardiovasc Imaging Rep. 2022;15(4):29–36.
9. Sharifrazi D, Alizadehsani R, Joloudari JH, Band SS, Hussain S, Sani ZA, et al. CNN-KCL: automatic myocarditis diagnosis using convolutional neural network combined with k-means clustering. Math Biosci Eng. 2022;19(3):2381–402.
10. Sharifrazi DAR, Joloudari JH, Band SS, Hussain S, Sani ZA, Hasanzadeh F, Shoeibi A, Dehzangi A, Sookhak M, Alinejad-Rokny H. CNN-KCL: automatic myocarditis diagnosis using convolutional neural network combined with k-means clustering. Math Biosci Eng. 2022;19(3):2381–402.
11. Karaboga D, Basturk B. On the performance of artificial bee colony (ABC) algorithm. Appl Soft Comput. 2008;8(1):687–97.
12. Baeßler B, Treutlein M, Schaarschmidt F, Stehning C, Schnackenburg B, Michels G, et al. A novel multiparametric imaging approach to acute myocarditis using T2-mapping and CMR feature tracking. J Cardiovasc Magn Reson. 2017;19(1):71.
13. Choi HM, Kim KH, Lee JM, Yoon YE, Lee SP, Park EA, et al. Myocardial fibrosis progression on cardiac magnetic resonance in hypertrophic cardiomyopathy. Heart. 2015;101(11):870–6.
14. Eckstein J, Moghadasi N, Körperich H, Akkuzu R, Sciacca V, Sohns C, et al. Machine-learning-based diagnostics of cardiac sarcoidosis using multi-Chamber Wall motion analyses. Diagnostics. 2023;13(14):2426.
15. Leiner T, Rueckert D, Suinesiaputra A, Baeßler B, Nezafat R, Išgum I, et al. Machine learning in cardiovascular magnetic resonance: basic concepts and applications. J Cardiovasc Magn Reson. 2019;21(1):61.
16. Singh M, Kumar A, Khanna NN, Laird JR, Nicolaides A, Faa G, et al. Artificial intelligence for cardiovascular disease risk assessment in personalised framework: a scoping review. EClinicalMedicine. 2024:73.
17. Haq I-U, Haq I, Xu B. Artificial intelligence in personalized cardiovascular medicine and cardiovascular imaging. Cardiovasc Diagn Ther. 2021;11(3):911.
18. Salih A, Boscolo Galazzo I, Gkontra P, Lee AM, Lekadir K, Raisi-Estabragh Z, et al. Explainable artificial intelligence and cardiac imaging: toward more interpretable models. Circ Cardiovasc Imaging. 2023;16(4):e014519.
19. Guleria P, Naga Srinivasu P, Ahmed S, Almusallam N, Alarfaj FK. XAI framework for cardiovascular disease prediction using classification techniques. Electronics. 2022;11(24):4086.
20. Blauwet LA, Cooper LT. Myocarditis. Prog Cardiovasc Dis. 2010;52(4):274–88.
21. Monney PLD, Muzzarelli S, Hullin R, Jeanrenaud X, Schwitter J. Imagerie de référence dans le diagnostic de la myocardite aiguë? [Cardiac magnetic resonance in acute myocarditis: a new non-invasive diagnostic gold standard?]. Rev Med Suisse. 2012;8(343):1177–83.
22. Caforio AL, Pankuweit S, Arbustini E, Basso C, Gimeno-Blanes J, Felix SB, et al. Current state of knowledge on aetiology, diagnosis, management, and therapy of myocarditis: a position statement of the European Society of Cardiology Working Group on myocardial and pericardial diseases. Eur Heart J. 2013;34(33):2636–48.
23. Łajczak PM, Jóźwik K. Artificial intelligence and myocarditis—a systematic review of current applications. Heart Fail Rev. 2024;1-18
24. Ferreira VM, Piechnik SK, Dall'Armellina E, Karamitsos TD, Francis JM, Ntusi N, et al. T1 mapping for the diagnosis of acute myocarditis using CMR: comparison to T2-weighted and late gadolinium enhanced imaging. JACC Cardiovasc Imaging. 2013;6(10):1048–58.
25. Georgiopoulos G, Figliozzi S, Sanguineti F, Aquaro GD, di Bella G, Stamatelopoulos K, et al. Prognostic impact of late gadolinium enhancement by cardiovascular magnetic resonance in myocarditis: a systematic review and meta-analysis. Circ Cardiovasc Imaging. 2021;14(1):e011492.
26. Catalano O, Antonaci S, Opasich C, Moro G, Mussida M, Perotti M, et al. Intra-observer and interobserver reproducibility of right ventricle volumes, function and mass by cardiac magnetic resonance. J Cardiovasc Med. 2007;8(10):807–14.
27. Alizadehsani R, Zangooei MH, Hosseini MJ, Habibi J, Khosravi A, Roshanzamir M, et al. Coronary artery disease detection using computational intelligence methods. Knowl Based Syst. 2016;109:187–97.
28. Nasarian E, Abdar M, Fahami MA, Alizadehsani R, Hussain S, Basiri ME, et al. Association between work-related features and coronary artery disease: a heterogeneous hybrid feature selection integrated with balancing approach. Pattern Recogn Lett. 2020;133:33–40.
29. Luetkens JA, Faron A, Isaak A, Dabir D, Kuetting D, Feisst A, et al. Comparison of original and 2018 Lake Louise criteria for diagnosis of acute myocarditis: results of a validation cohort. Radiol Cardiothorac Imaging. 2019;1(3):e190010.
30. Eichhorn C, Greulich S, Bucciarelli-Ducci C, Sznitman R, Kwong Raymond Y, Gräni C. Multiparametric cardiovascular magnetic resonance approach in diagnosing, monitoring, and prognostication of myocarditis. JACC Cardiovasc Imaging. 2022;15(7):1325–38.

31. Ferreira Vanessa M, Schulz-Menger J, Holmvang G, Kramer Christopher M, Carbone I, Sechtem U, et al. Cardiovascular magnetic resonance in nonischemic myocardial inflammation. J Am Coll Cardiol. 2018;72(24):3158–76.
32. Böttcher B, Beller E, Busse A, Cantré D, Yücel S, Öner A, et al. Fully automated quantification of left ventricular volumes and function in cardiac MRI: clinical evaluation of a deep learning-based algorithm. Int J Cardiovasc Imaging. 2020;36:2239–47.
33. kun Zhu Q. A novel method for myocardial image classification using data augmentation. Int J Adv Comput Sci Appl. 2023;14(6)
34. Cuadros J, Dugarte N, Wong S, Vanegas P, Morocho V, Medina R. ECG multilead QT interval estimation using support vector machines. J Healthc Eng. 2019;2019(1):6371871.
35. Cavallo AU, Di Donna C, Troisi J, Cerimele C, Cesareni M, Chiocchi M, et al. Radiomics analysis of short tau inversion recovery images in cardiac magnetic resonance for the prediction of late gadolinium enhancement in patients with acute myocarditis. Magn Reson Imaging. 2022;94:168–73.
36. Rahman SSMM, Chen Z, Lalande A, Decourselle T, Cochet A, Pommier T, et al. Automatic classification of patients with myocardial infarction or myocarditis based only on clinical data: a quick response. PLoS One. 2023;18(5):e0285165.
37. Puntmann VO, Zeiher AM, Nagel E. T1 and T2 mapping in myocarditis: seeing beyond the horizon of Lake Louise criteria and histopathology. Expert Rev Cardiovasc Ther. 2018;16(5):319–30.
38. Hinojar R, Foote L, Ucar EA, Dabir D, Schnackenburg B, Higgins DM, et al. Myocardial T2 mapping for improved detection of inflammatory myocardial involvement in acute and chronic myocarditis. J Cardiovasc Magn Reson. 2014;16
39. Canuti E, Toupin S, Sanguineti F, Hovasse T, Garot P, Champagne S, et al. Artificial intelligence fully automated assessment of global longitudinal strain predicts death in patients undergoing stress CMR. Arch Cardiovasc Dis. 2024;117(1):S57–S8.
40. Di Noto T, von Spiczak J, Mannil M, Gantert E, Soda P, Manka R, et al. Radiomics for distinguishing myocardial infarction from myocarditis at late gadolinium enhancement at MRI: comparison with subjective visual analysis. Radiol Cardiothorac Imaging. 2019;1(5):e180026.
41. Baessler B, Luecke C, Lurz J, Klingel K, von Roeder M, de Waha S, Besler C, Maintz D, Gutberlet M, Thiele H, Lurz P. Cardiac MRI texture analysis of T1 and T2 maps in patients with Infarctlike acute myocarditis. Radiology. 2018 nov;289(2):357–65.
42. Chou F-S, Ghimire LV. Identification of prognostic factors for pediatric myocarditis with a random forests algorithm-assisted approach. Pediatr Res. 2021;90(2):427–30.
43. Chou F-S, Ghimire LV. Machine learning for mortality prediction in pediatric myocarditis. Front Pediatr. 2021;9:644922.
44. Stephens AF, Šeman M, Diehl A, Pilcher D, Barbaro RP, Brodie D, et al. ECMO PAL: using deep neural networks for survival prediction in venoarterial extracorporeal membrane oxygenation. Intensive Care Med. 2023;49(9):1090–9.
45. Barker J, Li X, Khavandi S, Koeckerling D, Mavilakandy A, Pepper C, et al. Machine learning in sudden cardiac death risk prediction: a systematic review. Europace. 2022;24(11):1777–87.
46. Ali-Ahmed F, Dalgaard F, Al-Khatib SM. Sudden cardiac death in patients with myocarditis: evaluation, risk stratification, and management. Am Heart J. 2020;220:29–40.
47. Cremer PC, Klein AL, Imazio M. Diagnosis, risk stratification, and treatment of pericarditis: a review. JAMA. 2024;
48. Antonopoulos AS, Vrettos A, Androulakis E, Kamperou C, Vlachopoulos C, Tsioufis K, et al. Cardiac magnetic resonance imaging of pericardial diseases: a comprehensive guide. Eur Heart J Cardiovasc Imaging. 2023;24(8):983–98.
49. Sengupta PP, Huang Y-M, Bansal M, Ashrafi A, Fisher M, Shameer K, et al. Cognitive machine-learning algorithm for cardiac imaging: a pilot study for differentiating constrictive pericarditis from restrictive cardiomyopathy. Circ Cardiovasc Imaging. 2016;9(6):e004330.
50. Liu Y-L, Lin C-S, Cheng C-C, Lin C. A deep learning algorithm for detecting acute pericarditis by electrocardiogram. J Pers Med. 2022;12(7):1150.
51. Knockaert DC. Cardiac involvement in systemic inflammatory diseases. Eur Heart J. 2007;28(15):1797–804.
52. Aitken M, Davidson M, Chan MV, Urzua Fresno C, Vasquez LI, Huo YR, et al. Prognostic value of cardiac MRI and FDG PET in cardiac sarcoidosis: a systematic review and meta-analysis. Radiology. 2023;307(2):e222483.
53. Luo S, Dou WQ, Schoepf UJ, Varga-Szemes A, Pridgen WT, Zhang LJ. Cardiovascular magnetic resonance imaging in myocardial involvement of systemic lupus erythematosus. Trends Cardiovasc Med. 2023;33(6):346–54.
54. Ceccarelli F, Natalucci F, Picciariello L, Ciancarella C, Dolcini G, Gattamelata A, et al. Application of machine learning models in systemic lupus erythematosus. Int J Mol Sci. 2023;24(5):4514.
55. Lu C, Wang YG, Zaman F, Wu X, Adhaduk M, Chang A, et al. Predicting adverse cardiac events in sarcoidosis: deep learning from automated characterization of regional myocardial remodeling. Int J Cardiovasc Imaging. 2022;38(8):1825–36.
56. Shade JK, Prakosa A, Popescu DM, Yu R, Okada DR, Chrispin J, et al. Predicting risk of sudden cardiac death in patients with cardiac sarcoidosis using multimodality imaging and personalized heart modeling in a multivariable classifier. Sci Adv. 2021;7(31):eabi8020.
57. Lanera C, Berchialla P, Sharma A, Minto C, Gregori D, Baldi I. Screening PubMed abstracts: is class

imbalance always a challenge to machine learning? Syst Rev. 2019;8(1):317.
58. Rao RS, Dewangan S, Mishra A, Gupta M. A study of dealing class imbalance problem with machine learning methods for code smell severity detection using PCA-based feature selection technique. Sci Rep. 2023;13(1):16245.
59. Hufnagel G, Pankuweit S, Richter A, Schönian U, Maisch B. The European study of epidemiology and treatment of cardiac inflammatory diseases (ESETCID).First epidemiological results. Herz. 2000;25(3):279–85.

7 SWOT Analysis of the Integration of MRI in Cardiology: Strengths, Weaknesses, Opportunities, and Threats

Amir Ghaffari Jolfayi, Mahshad Sarikhani, Aryan Aarabi, Hamidreza Ghasemirad, Zahra Dehghanian, and Mohammadhossein Mozafarybazargany

Abstract

This chapter explores the transformative role of Artificial Intelligence (AI) in enhancing Cardiac Magnetic Resonance Imaging (CMR) and its integration in cardiology, analyzed through a comprehensive SWOT framework, examining its strengths, weaknesses, opportunities, and threats. AI has revolutionized CMR by improving diagnostic precision, reducing acquisition times, enabling non-contrast imaging, and automating workflows, thus enhancing accessibility and patient comfort. CMR, recognized as the gold-standard imaging modality for its tissue characterization and functional assessment capabilities, significantly impacts clinical outcomes in cardiovascular disease management.

However, the adoption of CMR faces challenges, including high costs, technological complexity, limited accessibility, and the need for specialized training. These factors restrict its broader use, particularly in low-resource settings. Patient cooperation, prolonged scan times, and contraindications with certain implanted devices add further practical hurdles.

Opportunities abound in AI-enhanced imaging, enabling personalized diagnostics, superior prognostic capabilities, and precision

Authors Amir Ghaffari Jolfayi and Mahshad Sarikhani have contributed equality and shared the first co-authorship.

The original version of the chapter has been revised. A correction to this chapter can be found at https://doi.org/10.1007/978-981-95-0313-1_9

A. Ghaffari Jolfayi
Cardiovascular Imaging Research Center, Rajaie Cardiovascular Institute, Iran University of Medical Sciences, Tehran, Iran

M. Sarikhani
Department of Radiology, Shariati Hospital, Tehran University of Medical Sciences, Tehran, Iran

A. Aarabi
School of Medicine, Shahid Beheshti University of Medical Sciences, Tehran, Iran

H. Ghasemirad
Student Research Committee, Shahid Sadoughi University of Medical Sciences, Yazd, Iran

Z. Dehghanian
Department of Computer Engineering, Sharif University of Technology, Tehran, Iran

M. Mozafarybazargany (✉)
Cardiovascular Imaging Research Center, Rajaie Cardiovascular Institute, Iran University of Medical Sciences, Tehran, Iran

Cardiovascular Research Center, Rajaie Cardiovascular Institute, Tehran, Iran

A. Ghaffari Jolfayi (ed.), *Navigating Cardiology's Future*, https://doi.org/10.1007/978-981-95-0313-1_7

medicine approaches in cardiology. Yet, CMR's position is increasingly challenged by advancements in competing modalities such as CT and echocardiography, coupled with ethical, regulatory, and technological barriers to AI integration.

This chapter emphasizes the necessity for innovation and cross-sector collaboration to overcome these challenges, ensuring that AI-enhanced CMR continues to evolve and maintain its pivotal role in the future of cardiac imaging and healthcare delivery.

Keywords

Cardiac magnetic resonance imaging · Strengths · Weaknesses · Opportunities · Threats · Deep learning · Machine learning · Artificial intelligence

Cardiac Magnetic Resonance Imaging (CMR) has emerged as a cornerstone in cardiology, offering unparalleled precision in diagnosing and managing cardiovascular diseases. With advancements in Artificial Intelligence (AI), CMR is transforming into a faster, more accessible, and highly accurate imaging modality, pushing the boundaries of personalized medicine. However, its integration into routine clinical practice faces challenges. This chapter examines the strengths, weaknesses, opportunities, and threats of AI-enhanced CMR, shedding light on its current capabilities and future potential in shaping cardiovascular care.

7.1 Strengths

7.1.1 Strength of Cardiac Magnetic Resonance Imaging

CMR has been selected as the gold standard of diagnosis in various cardiovascular diseases due to its tissue characterization capability, excellent ventricular and valvular function identification, and anatomical evaluation [1, 2]. This detailed information is not to be elicited through other imaging modalities, at least with the details offered by CMR [2]. Utilization of Late Gadolinium Enhancement (LGE) CMR in the diagnostic approach of cardiomyopathies has been reported to alter the diagnosis and considerably impact clinical management [1]. Taking the value of the timely diagnosis of cardiomyopathies into account, CMR would improve the prognosis of these patients. It promptly enables Implantable Cardioverter-Defibrillator (ICD) or medical therapy initiation, contributing to improved clinical outcomes [1]. Preliminary studies have found that CMR reduces the cost of cardiomyopathy for patients; however, large-scale studies have yet to assess the cost-effectiveness of CMR in this patient population [1].

CMR impacted the diagnosis of nearly half of the patients subjected to CMR for Heart Failure (HF) [1]. In addition to the diagnostic value of CMR in various cardiac diseases, it is also invaluable in prognostic evaluation. For instance, it unraveled an unrecognized pathology linked to poor prognosis in more than one-fourth of HF with Preserved Ejection Fraction (HFpEF) patients [1].

7.1.2 Integrating Artificial Intelligence with CMR

The initial use of AI in medicine dates back to 1976 and has been growing extensively since [3]. AI is employed in cardiac imaging, especially CMR. It has shown enhancement in acquisition, measurement, and interpretation, and offers a substitute to the contrast agent CMR [4–8].

Low special resolution CMR acquisition integrated with AI reconstruction reduces the acquisition time by nearly half. It improves patient convenience by reducing breath-holding time, leaving the quality and volumetric data unaffected compared to normal resolution CMR [4]. A deep learning convoluted neural network model performed a quality assessment of three-dimensional whole-heart CMR, with results comparable to those of experts [9]. Reconstruction and noise reduction AI models have also been used to improve the quality of CMR LGE images. The noise reduction model could successfully improve image quality in ischemic cardiomyopathy patients [10].

Another utility of AI models for enhanced CMR acquisition is the proposed AI model assessing the quality of LGE CMR in real-time. In LGE CMR reporting, uncertainty often arises in differentiating LGE from an artifact. The proposed AI model could detect the potential uncertainty, enabling further acquisition or repetition during scan acquisition [11].

While LGE imaging offers substantial information in a wide range of cardiac diseases, it is contraindicated in renal impairment, and there has been growing concern regarding its accumulation within extracardiac tissues [6–8]. Considering the fact that one of the invaluable capabilities of CMR, tissue characterization, relies on LGE for optimal results, a growing body of evidence is trying to substitute the need for LGE with integrating AI into non-contrast CMR [6, 7]. A deep learning model developed by Zhang et al. aimed to detect chronic Myocardial Infarction (MI) using cine CMR showed noninferiority to LGE CMR, even for transmurality, segment, and area delineation of the MI [8]. CMR Virtual Native Enhancement (VNE) has been introduced as an AI-enhanced CMR with the potential to substitute LGE CMR without a contrast agent. VNE attained better image quality than LGE, with non-inferior lesion quantification and distribution [12].

CMR interpretation is time-consuming and has far-from-perfect inter- and intra-observer variability [13]. Taking advantage of AI models' ability to recognize patterns in detailed and high-level information, efforts have been made to assist, facilitate, and enhance CMR interpretation [13].

In a large study on 9719 patients evaluating 11 cardiovascular diseases, an AI-enhanced CMR attained excellent performance in screening and diagnosis of cardiovascular diseases, outperforming cardiologists in pulmonary arterial hypertension diagnosis [5]. AI-enhanced CMR enables taking undefined CMR features into account [5]. Non-contrast CMR is suggested to accurately identify Hypertrophic Cardiomyopathy (HCM) patients without scars using a deep learning model. This model could be employed for screening purposes, reducing the need for LGE CMR in HCM patients [14].

Integrating strain analysis through feature tracking, volume-based temporal variations, and three-dimensional structural analysis derived from CMR into the AI model enables incremental prognostic value in post-MI patients, enhancing risk assessment and patient management [15]. The prognostic role of AI-enhanced CMR is not confined to MI patients. AI-enhanced LGE CMR showed incremental predictive strength for ventricular arrhythmia risk stratification of systolic dysfunction without ischemia. Considering the fatality of ventricular arrhythmias in this patient population, AI-enhanced LGE CMR could potentially improve patient outcomes [16]. AI-enhanced LGE CMR also exhibited additive predictive value for all-cause mortality prediction in cardiac amyloidosis, improving risk stratification [17]. These models even outperformed models based on the current guidelines regarding ICD implantation with accurate myocardial scar quantification [18].

7.2 Weaknesses

Despite advanced features, CMR presents various challenges that limit its broader application in routine clinical practice. These challenges include high costs, accessibility issues, technological constraints, and the need for specialized training. The following will explore these limitations in detail, providing a comprehensive understanding of the factors hindering CMR adoption.

7.2.1 Technological Complexity and Procedural Challenges

CMR is technically demanding, requiring longer scan times than other imaging modalities. The average scan duration ranges from 30 minutes to an hour, during which patients must remain unmoved and perform breath-hold sequences to ensure image clarity. This can be problematic for patients with arrhythmias, respiratory issues, or those who cannot tolerate enclosed spaces (Claustrophobia) or pediatric patients, leading to artifacts that degrade image quality. For instance, irregular heart rhythms or those unable to do breath-holding for extended periods may produce suboptimal images that limit the diagnostic value of the scan [19, 20].

Moreover, the acquisition process for CMR involves various complex sequences, such as T1 and T2 mapping, phase-contrast imaging, and LGE. These sequences require precise synchronization with the patient's cardiac cycle, which arrhythmias can disrupt. While real-time cine MRI is being developed to address this limitation, it remains a trade-off between spatiotemporal resolution and scan time, making it an incomplete solution [21].

7.2.2 Accessibility and Equipment Availability

In high-income countries, the demand for CMR has been steadily increasing. However, many healthcare facilities continue to face significant limitations due to the availability of MRI scanners, which are essential for conducting these exams. A notable example is the United Kingdom, where the demand for CMR scans surged 253% between 2008 and 2013. Despite this marked increase, the supply of MRI scanners and the availability of trained personnel have not grown at the same rate, leading to challenges in meeting the rising demand [22]. The insufficient number of available scanners often results in long patient waiting times, diagnosis delays, and increased pressure on healthcare systems to optimize existing resources. This imbalance between demand and supply illustrates a critical bottleneck in providing CMR services in even the most resource-rich settings.

The situation is even more challenging in low- to middle-income countries, where the cost of acquiring, maintaining, and operating CMR equipment can be prohibitively expensive. In these regions, the lack of financial resources compounds the difficulty in accessing advanced imaging technologies, such as CMR, which are crucial for accurate cardiovascular diagnoses. Although there has been growing interest in the potential of using lower field strength (0.55T) MRI scanners as a more affordable option to enhance accessibility, these alternatives come with their own set of challenges. Lower-field strength scanners generally produce reduced-quality images and require longer acquisition times, which may compromise their utility in clinical practice [21]. This disparity in access to high-quality imaging technology is one of the most significant barriers to the widespread adoption of CMR, especially in regions where healthcare resources are already constrained. Addressing this gap remains a key challenge for ensuring equitable access to advanced diagnostic tools globally.

7.2.3 Cost and Financial Barriers

The high cost of CMR is another major limitation to its broader use. Without insurance, a standard CMR in the United States can range from **$1000 to $5000**, making it one of the most expensive cardiac imaging modalities. This is significantly higher compared to the cost of other imaging techniques like echocardiography (**$400 to $1500**) or Single Photon Emission Computed Tomography (SPECT) (**$500 to $1500**). While CMR is a non-invasive procedure offering intricate functional and anatomical information, its high cost restricts its use to specific cases where other imaging modalities are insufficient.

Indirect costs further elevate the financial burden associated with CMR. These include the need for highly specialized team members, such as radiologists and technologists trained in cardiac imaging, as well as the high maintenance and operational costs of the MRI scanner. Additionally, frequent software updates and hardware advancements add to the overall expenses [19, 21]. For many healthcare systems, the combination of high upfront costs and the continuous expenses of operating CMR make it less feasible to use routinely, even in advanced cardiac centers.

Despite the high upfront costs, studies have shown that CMR can be cost-effective in certain high-risk populations, e.g., suspected Coronary Artery Disease (CAD), where its diagnostic accuracy can prevent unnecessary invasive procedures. However, its cost-effectiveness is limited to specific scenarios, making it less appealing for routine use in general patient populations [23, 24].

7.2.4 Training and Expertise Limitations

CMR is a highly specialized modality that demands a significant level of expertise from both physicians and technologists. Unlike other imaging techniques, such as echocardiography or Computed Tomography (CT) angiography, the interpretation of CMR scans is notably more complex and requires advanced knowledge. Even radiologists with extensive experience in other imaging modalities must undergo specific and targeted training in CMR to ensure accurate interpretation of these scans. This is particularly critical given the detailed anatomical and functional information that CMR provides, which is crucial for patient management and diagnosis. Additionally, the continuous evolution of CMR technology, with innovative techniques like T1 and T2 mapping, strain imaging, and Four-Dimensional (4D) flow imaging, further emphasizes the need for ongoing education and skill enhancement. These novel sequences offer deeper insights into cardiac pathology but require radiologists to remain up-to-date with the latest advancements to maximize their diagnostic utility [21, 25].

Training in CMR is not only time-intensive but also demands continuous education to keep pace with the rapidly evolving field. Given this modality's complexity and specialized nature, the learning curve can be steep, and maintaining proficiency requires regular exposure to CMR. Unfortunately, many physicians and technologists do not receive adequate hands-on training in CMR during their formal education, mainly due to the limited availability of this imaging technique in certain training programs. This issue is especially pronounced in smaller hospitals or regions where CMR is underutilized, leaving healthcare providers with insufficient practical experience to harness its diagnostic capabilities fully. As a result, CMR may be underutilized or misinterpreted, leading to suboptimal diagnostic outcomes and an inability to take full advantage of the modality's advanced potential. Bridging this gap in training and ensuring that healthcare professionals have access to adequate CMR education remains a key challenge in optimizing the use of this sophisticated imaging tool [20, 22].

7.2.5 Patient Factors and Practical Challenges

Another key limitation of CMR is its reliance on patient cooperation, which presents several practical challenges. The procedure typically requires patients to remain still for extended periods, as scan times generally range from 30 to 60 minutes. This extended duration can be problematic for specific individuals, particularly those who suffer from claustrophobia, anxiety, or respiratory difficulties. Maintaining stillness during the scan is critical for obtaining accurate images, and many protocols require breath-holding at specific intervals to enhance image clarity. Patients unable to hold their breaths consistently due to respiratory issues or other conditions may produce motion artifacts that significantly degrade the diagnostic quality of the images. This can lead to inconclusive results, requiring repeat imaging, which further strains resources and patient tolerance [21, 25].

Moreover, implanted devices, such as pacemakers or defibrillators, have been a contraindication for MRI due to safety risks associated with magnetic fields. While recent technological advancements have allowed patients with MRI-conditional devices to undergo CMR, there are still notable limitations. Many healthcare facilities are not yet equipped with the specialized protocols or the appropriate infrastructure to safely manage these cases, restricting access to this advanced diagnostic tool for a subset of patients.

This gap in capability, despite technological advancements, represents a significant barrier to broader patient accessibility to CMR, as not all centers have the necessary expertise or resources to accommodate patients with complex medical devices [21].

7.3 Summary of Key Limitations

While CMR is an invaluable tool for detailed cardiovascular imaging, offering superior soft-tissue contrast and functional analysis, its widespread adoption is hindered by several significant limitations. The high cost of the equipment and procedure, limited accessibility, and the need for specialized training all contribute to its restricted use. Furthermore, the technological complexity of CMR, the prolonged scan times in addition to patients' waiting times, and patient-related factors such as claustrophobia and inability to hold breath during scans pose practical challenges that reduce its feasibility in routine clinical practice. As technology advances and accessibility improves, these limitations may be mitigated. Still, for now, CMR remains a specialized tool that is most useful in select cases where other imaging modalities cannot provide sufficient diagnostic information [19, 20, 22].

7.4 Opportunities

CMR non-invasively evaluates the structure and function of the heart, and it has become widely accepted as a useful diagnostic tool for cardiovascular disease [26, 27]. The development of AI, mainly through neural networks and deep learning, has significantly improved the prospects for individualized heart disease management in medical imaging, especially MRI. These technologies automate post-processing, enhance diagnostic accuracy, and deliver more reliable results [28–30]. Concerning these features, Machine Learning (ML) algorithms, as well as advanced MRI systems, use predictive analysis to create more accurate, customized treatment modalities specific to every individual patient. This individualization not only incorporates resources for the provision of probable diagnosis but also aids health practitioners in harnessing such resources to prevent diseases before they become more serious. As such systems include genomic data, Electronic Health Records (EHR), and continuous monitoring parameters, they present a comprehensive picture of the patient, which enhances clinical management and expedites treatment.

Additionally, these features of AI-based MRI represent a trend toward real-time measurement of the target, achieving immediate interpretations of images with higher accuracy. Quick interpretation is essential in identifying minor changes that can be missed by standard imaging evaluation, enabling timely treatment, which can result in improved outcomes. In addition to that, the inclusion of AI not only reduces manual effort by automating repetitive tasks but also enhances the interpretation of medical images. This minimizes variability and increases the likelihood of accurate diagnoses. While analyzing the multitude of possibilities posed by the enhanced MRI, including the effect of AI, it becomes evident that these advancements do not only improve the accuracy of diagnosis and prognosis; they redefine the future of cardiology, enabling a better approach toward personalized medicine, improving patient care and the healthcare delivery system.

7.4.1 Opportunities for Personalized Cardiac Care

One of the most compelling opportunities presented by AI-enhanced MRI is the ability to plan personalized management strategies tailored to the unique characteristics of each patient. AI's proficiency in predictive analytics allows for forecasting potential health issues based on historical data, which facilitates early detection and treatment. This enables risk identification before it develops into severe illnesses, resulting in the timely implementation of preventive healthcare measures [31–40]. AI can personalize medicine by enabling customized diagnostic strategies and treatment plans. This leads to improved diagnostic precision and more tailored treatment regimens, which improves the level of individualization in healthcare [41].

AI also provides extensive health insights through its integration with additional technologies, such as EHRs. By offering a holistic picture of the medical history and current status of the patient, this integration not only enhances clinical decision-making but also expedites patient care [42]. Furthermore, AI enables a more comprehensive healthcare approach and clinical decision-making by combining various patient data sources, including genomic data and medical imaging, facilitating the development of customized management strategies, more accurate risk assessments, and therapeutic response tracking [43].

7.4.2 Rapid Assessment of MRI Scans

AI could evaluate medical images quickly and accurately. This capability aids in identifying diseases that may be difficult to detect in their early stages using conventional methods. Early identification is essential, as it can lead to timely interventions that save lives and enhance treatment success [44–46]. AI applications have greatly improved the efficiency of image acquisition and analysis in CMR. For instance, neural networks can reconstruct an MRI from expeditiously captured under-sampled data throughout various sequences. One notable achievement includes a super-resolution CMR angiography system based on deep learning, which has enabled the reconstruction of low-resolution data scanned in just 50 seconds, resulting in a 16-fold increase in acquisition speed while maintaining comparable quantitative and perceptible image quality to higher-resolution imaging [47]. The suggested technique achieved a 16-fold increase in acquisition time while maintaining comparable perceptible and quantitative quality to the 1.2 mm high-resolution image. Similar outcomes, surpassing compressed sensing reconstruction in CMR angiography 1.2 mm acquisition by 9 times, have been obtained with an undersampled multi-scale variational neural network reconstruction [48]. Steeden et al. [49] performed super-resolution reconstruction on low-resolution three-dimensional whole heart balanced Steady State Free Precession (bSSFP) datasets using the Three-Dimensional (3D) residual U-net, a convolutional neural network. This resulted in diagnostic confidence and accuracy for congestive heart failure cases that was comparable to that of whole heart bSSFP obtained in high-resolution.

7.4.3 Improving Diagnostic Accuracy

Improving diagnosis accuracy is crucial for efficient treatment and positive clinical outcomes in modern medicine, especially cardiology. With the introduction of AI-enhanced MRI technology, diagnostic imaging has seen a dramatic change that has opened the door for novel strategies that improve image interpretation, include multi-modal data, and allow predictive modeling. The advancement in diagnostic skills not only tackles the intricacies of heart disorders but also promotes more preemptive and customized patient care.

7.4.4 Enhanced Prognostic Accuracy

AI can assess MRI results in conjunction with longitudinal health data to forecast the future progression and outcome of diseases. In one study utilizing principal component analysis, 3D right ventricular cardiac motion was used as an input to predict the four-year survival of pulmonary hypertension. In addition to right-sided heart catheterization-derived features and clinical, functional, and regular characteristics, this method demonstrated an AUC of 0.73 for integrating 3D-CMR features in the algorithm (AUC 0.60 without 3D-CMR features) [50]. In another study of tetralogy of Fallot patients subjected to repair, a predictive algorithm (AUC 0.87 for substantial deterioration) evaluating decreased Left Ventricular (LV) function demonstrated that AI models could enable timely intervention planning for patients at higher risk [51].

7.4.5 Potential Technical Advantages

AI models are going to address several limitations associated with CMR, particularly its time-consuming image acquisition and complex post-processing requirements. AI algorithms have been developed to accelerate image acquisition, potentially reducing scan times to just a few minutes [52]. Additionally, AI-driven software can automate the segmentation of the heart's chambers and blood vessels, reducing the reliance on manual interpretation and making the process more consistent and less operator-dependent [53].

AI can also enhance CMR's diagnostic accuracy by identifying patterns that may not be visible to the human eye. It is going to design AI models that can assist in detecting subtle myocardial fibrosis or early signs of cardiomyopathy, improving early diagnosis and patient outcomes. Moreover, AI has the potential to predict clinical outcomes based on CMR data, aiding in treatment planning and risk stratification [54].

7.4.6 Future Perspectives

To determine if ML approaches are useful in clinical practice, controlled prospective clinical trials comparing ML techniques with human evaluation of magnetic resonance datasets are required. Other cohorts, such as data from various centers and acquisition devices, must be used to validate the algorithms in addition to the one under consideration. Additionally, assessing each algorithm's effectiveness on a shared dataset is crucial for comparing how well they perform in relation to one another. For this field to advance, publicly available software would be necessary for other parties to run, examine, and alter the program, allowing them to make improvements and keep an eye out for any potential bias in the algorithm [55].

AI in CMR is an innovative development that improves cardiovascular care and is critical in management decisions. Since AI ensures correct image analysis and combines other aspects of data, it helps healthcare practitioners create an individualized approach and treatment options for their patients. The use of real-time data and predictive analytics is also instrumental in the management and follow-up of patients, as well as in predicting the course of a disease and accordingly planning for possible treatment. As such, the technological advancements in healthcare, particularly these sophisticated innovations, hold immense potential. When implemented effectively, they pave the way for improved patient outcomes through more targeted and focused care, offering a promising prospect. This will, in the long run, contribute to the evolution of how cardiovascular diseases will be treated.

7.5 Threats: Competing Modalities and AI Adoption Barriers

CMR has long been considered one of the most advanced imaging modalities in cardiology due to its detailed structural and functional imaging capabilities, as well as its ability to provide non-invasive tissue characterization without exposing patients to ionizing radiation [56]. However, despite its superiority in certain applications, CMR faces increasing competition from other imaging modalities, as well as challenges in adopting AI technologies that could further enhance its clinical utility [57]. In this part, we will explore the potential threats to CMR's dominance in the field of cardiology, focusing on the rise of alternative imaging modalities and the barriers to AI adoption.

7.5.1 Artificial Intelligence in Cardiac Imaging: Potential and Barriers

AI holds significant potential to enhance the capabilities of CMR by improving image acquisition, analysis, and interpretation [58]. AI, especially deep learning, is developing to automate image segmentation, detect abnormalities, and predict clinical outcomes more accurately than traditional methods. However, the adoption of AI in MRI is not without challenges [59].

7.5.1.1 Data Quality and Availability

One of the major barriers to AI adoption in CMR is the need for high-quality, standardized training data. AI models require large datasets to train effectively, but CMR data are often fragmented, with variations in imaging protocols, scanner specifications, and patient demographics across institutions [60]. This lack of standardization makes it difficult to develop generalizable AI models that could be applicable in most clinical settings [61].

7.5.1.2 Robustness and Reproducibility Across Diverse Populations

A critical aspect to highlight here is the concept of robustness, a hot topic in AI. Robustness refers to the ability of an AI model to perform reliably across diverse and unseen scenarios. In addition, the results obtained from an AI model should be reproducible. In clinical applications, robustness becomes even more crucial due to the potential for catastrophic outcomes and severely adverse results if these considerations are not adequately addressed. Ensuring that AI systems are both robust and generalizable is essential for their safe and effective integration into routine clinical practice [62].

7.5.1.3 Regulatory and Ethical Challenges

The clinical implication of AI raises several regulatory and ethical concerns. AI-driven algorithms are subject to strict regulatory approval processes, which can delay their integration into routine clinical workflows [63]. Moreover, the "black box" nature of AI, i.e., the concealed process of decision-making, provokes ethical concerns regarding responsibility and trust in AI-driven diagnoses [64].

An additional issue that warrants attention is the management of patient data used for training AI algorithms. Patients must provide explicit consent for using their medical images, and mechanisms must be in place to honor their right to revoke consent at any time. If a patient withdraws their consent, ensuring their data can be efficiently and securely removed from the training dataset becomes critical. Here, implementing differential privacy techniques can play a crucial role, as they allow AI systems to learn from data without retaining identifiable information, thereby addressing ethical and practical challenges in managing patient data [65, 66].

7.5.1.4 Black Box Image Interpretation

Although the integration of AI and CMR opens up novel and intriguing opportunities to facilitate post-processing and improve diagnostic accuracy, most of the AI-based diagnostic tools work based on a black box. Through the automation of scan planning and acquisition parameter selection, as well as accelerated acquisition and post-processing, the employment of AI greatly expedites the examination workflow. Still, there are many concerns about the decisions made by AI or deep learning algorithms due to the black box and unclear nature of the decisions. Many of these AI-based tools are in a black-box mode, lacking inherent interpretability and requiring additional effort to make their workings understandable, which should be considered in designing future models [67–69].

7.5.1.5 Resistance to Change

Clinicians' resistance to adopting AI technologies is another significant barrier. Many clinicians are hesitant to rely on AI for critical diagnostic decisions, fearing that AI may replace human expertise or lead to incorrect diagnoses [70]. Some concerns pertain to the black-box nature of AI models, while most can be attributed to conflicts of interest and job threats. Integrating AI into CMR will require substantial training and education to ensure clinicians understand how to use AI to augment, rather than replace, their expertise [71].

7.5.2 Advancements in Other Imaging Modalities and Their Competition with CMR

7.5.2.1 Competing Imaging Modalities: A Rising Challenge

Recently, imaging modalities other than CMR have made significant advancements, challenging CMR's position as the gold standard in various cardiology applications. These competing technologies, like nuclear imaging, CT, and echocardiography, offer unique strengths that could threaten MRI's role in clinical practice [72]. In addition, CT imaging, particularly coronary CT Angiography (CTA), has gained widespread popularity in cardiology due to its speed, accessibility, and ability to visualize coronary arteries with high accuracy. Unlike MRI, which is more time-consuming and costly, CT can provide rapid, detailed anatomical images, making it especially useful in emergency settings [73]. The advent of new-generation CT scanners with improved spatial resolution and lower radiation doses has significantly reduced the gap between CT and MRI in terms of safety and image quality [74]. For example, dual-energy CT and photon-counting CT systems can now provide advanced tissue characterization, narrowing the advantage that MRI traditionally held in soft tissue imaging [75].

CT's rapid image acquisition, particularly for CAD, makes it a serious competitor to CMR, especially in time-sensitive clinical scenarios where speed and accessibility are crucial [76]. Moreover, CT's increasing ability to visualize myocardial perfusion and tissue differentiation is encroaching upon MRI's previously uncontested areas, such as myocardial viability assessment [77].

7.5.2.2 Echocardiography: The Ubiquitous Workhorse

Echocardiography remains the most commonly used imaging modality in cardiology, given its cost-effectiveness, widespread availability, and portability [78]. Advancements in echocardiographic techniques, such as 3D echocardiography and strain analysis, have improved their ability to assess myocardial function and detect subtle abnormalities in heart motion [79].

While CMR provides superior tissue characterization, echocardiography excels in real-time bedside imaging and functional assessment [78]. Its portability and low cost make it the go-to modality in resource-limited settings, challenging CMR's relevance in routine diagnostic workups. Additionally, advances in software have made echocardiographic measurements more precise, particularly in assessing ejection fraction and wall motion abnormalities [80].

7.5.2.3 Nuclear Imaging and Hybrid Modalities

Nuclear imaging, including SPECT and Positron Emission Tomography (PET), provides a complementary assessment of myocardial perfusion and metabolism that CMR cannot easily offer [81]. These techniques are often used in conjunction with other modalities, such as CT or MRI, to give a broader perspective of both the structure and function of the heart [82]. Hybrid imaging, combining modalities like PET-MRI or SPECT-CT, is another growing area that threatens MRI's standalone dominance. Hybrid imaging offers clinicians simultaneous anatomical and functional assessment, reducing the need for multiple tests [83]. It is a compelling alternative to CMR, particularly in complex cases like ischemic heart disease, where detailed perfusion imaging and metabolic assessments are required [84].

7.6 The Future of MRI in Cardiology

While MRI remains a powerful tool in cardiac imaging, its continued dominance is far from guaranteed. Competing imaging modalities like CT and echocardiography, along with emerging hybrid techniques, offer distinct advantages that may make them preferable in certain clinical scenarios [85]. Although AI promises to transform MRI, its widespread adoption challenges must be addressed to incorporate it seamlessly into everyday clinical practice [61]. Using AI in

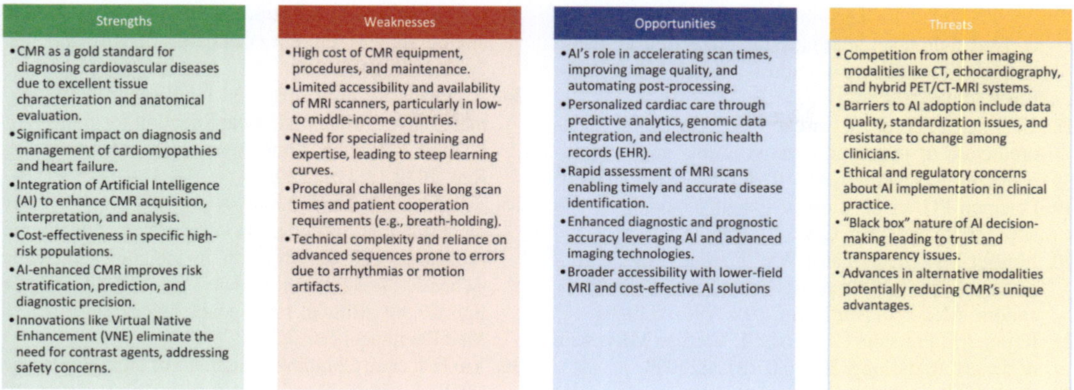

Fig. 7.1 SWOT analysis key point—application of AI in Cardiac Magnetic Resonance Imaging

cardiovascular imaging, particularly in specialized modalities like CMR, offers significant potential, especially in human-in-the-loop setups. It can greatly enhance efficiency and speed for doctors. However, we are still far from achieving standalone implementation, as it requires supervision due to its current limitations.

CMR must continue to evolve to overcome the challenges posed by these competing modalities and AI adoption barriers. The collaboration of AI developers with regulatory authorities and clinicians will be essential to ensure that AI is implemented safely and effectively in CMR (Fig. 7.1) [60].

References

1. Popa O-A, et al. Impact of cardiac magnetic resonance on the diagnosis and management of patients with cardiomyopathies choice. Roman J Cardiol. 2024;11:12.
2. Shah S, Chryssos ED, Parker H. Magnetic resonance imaging: a wealth of cardiovascular information. Ochsner J. 2009;9(4):266–77.
3. Mamedov M, Savchuk E, Karimov A. Artificial intelligence in cardiology. Artificial Intelligence (AI). 1255:0416.
4. Kravchenko D, et al. Deep learning super-resolution reconstruction for fast and high-quality cine cardiovascular magnetic resonance. Eur Radiol. 2024;
5. Wang YR, et al. Screening and diagnosis of cardiovascular disease using artificial intelligence-enabled cardiac magnetic resonance imaging. Nat Med. 2024;30(5):1471–80.
6. Howard, J.P. and H.C. Cheung, From gadolinium to generative AI: the quest for contrast-free cardiac imaging: Circ Cardiovasc Imaging, 2024. 17(9): p. e017361.
7. Cicek V, Bagci U. AI-powered contrast-free cardiovascular magnetic resonance imaging for myocardial infarction. Front Cardiovasc Med. 2024:11.
8. Zhang N, et al. Deep learning for diagnosis of chronic myocardial infarction on nonenhanced cardiac cine MRI. Radiology. 2019;291(3):606–17.
9. Piccini D, et al. Deep learning to automate reference-free image quality assessment of whole-heart MR images. Radiol Artif Intell. 2020;2(3):e190123.
10. Muscogiuri G, et al. Feasibility of late gadolinium enhancement (LGE) in ischemic cardiomyopathy using 2D-multisegment LGE combined with artificial intelligence reconstruction deep learning noise reduction algorithm. Int J Cardiol. 2021;343:164–70.
11. Zaman S, et al. Quality assurance of late gadolinium enhancement cardiac magnetic resonance images: a deep learning classifier for confidence in the presence or absence of abnormality with potential to prompt real-time image optimization. J Cardiovasc Magn Reson. 2024;26(1)
12. Zhang Q, et al. Toward replacing late gadolinium enhancement with artificial intelligence virtual native enhancement for gadolinium-free cardiovascular magnetic resonance tissue characterization in hypertrophic cardiomyopathy. Circulation. 2021;144(8):589–99.
13. Aromiwura AA, et al. The role of artificial intelligence in cardiovascular magnetic resonance imaging. Prog Cardiovasc Dis. 2024;86:13–25.
14. Fahmy AS, et al. Radiomics and deep learning for myocardial scar screening in hypertrophic cardiomyopathy. J Cardiovasc Magn Reson. 2022;24(1)
15. Corral Acero J, et al. Comprehensive characterization of cardiac contraction for improved post-infarction risk assessment. Sci Rep. 2024;14(1)
16. Kolk MZH, et al. Multimodal explainable artificial intelligence identifies patients with non-ischaemic cardiomyopathy at risk of lethal ventricular arrhythmias. Sci Rep. 2024;14(1)

17. Zhou XY, et al. Late gadolinium enhanced cardiac MR derived radiomics approach for predicting all-cause mortality in cardiac amyloidosis: a multicenter study. Eur Radiol. 2024;34(1):402–10.
18. Ghanbari F, et al. AI cardiac MRI scar analysis aids prediction of major arrhythmic events in the multicenter DERIVATE registry. Radiology. 2023;307(3)
19. Peterson PG, et al. Cardiac imaging modalities and appropriate use. Prim Care. 2018;45(1):155–68.
20. Pfeiffer MP, Biederman RWW. Cardiac MRI: a general overview with emphasis on current use and indications. Med Clin North Am. 2015;99(4):849–61.
21. Rajiah PS, François CJ, Leiner T. Cardiac MRI: state of the art. Radiology. 2023;307(3):e223008.
22. Ripley DP, et al. Cardiovascular magnetic resonance imaging: what the general cardiologist should know. Heart. 2016;102(19):1589–603.
23. Azari S, et al. Cost-effectiveness of cardiovascular magnetic resonance imaging compared to common strategies in the diagnosis of coronary artery disease: a systematic review. Heart Fail Rev. 2023;28(6):1357–82.
24. Centonze M, et al. Cardiac-CT and cardiac-MR cost-effectiveness: a literature review. Radiol Med. 2020;125(11):1200–7.
25. Busse A, et al. Cardiac MRI—Update 2020. Radiologe. 2020;60(1):33–40.
26. Messroghli DR, et al. Clinical recommendations for cardiovascular magnetic resonance mapping of T1, T2, T2* and extracellular volume: a consensus statement by the Society for Cardiovascular Magnetic Resonance (SCMR) endorsed by the European Association for Cardiovascular Imaging (EACVI). J Cardiovasc Magn Reson. 2016;19(1):75.
27. von Knobelsdorff-Brenkenhoff F, Schulz-Menger J. Role of cardiovascular magnetic resonance in the guidelines of the European Society of Cardiology. J Cardiovasc Magn Reson. 2016;18(1):6.
28. Wang G, et al. Image reconstruction is a new frontier of machine learning. IEEE Trans Med Imaging. 2018;37(6):1289–96.
29. Ben Yedder H, Cardoen B, Hamarneh G. Deep learning for biomedical image reconstruction: a survey. Artif Intell Rev. 2021;54(1):215–51.
30. Zhang H-M, Dong B. A review on deep learning in medical image reconstruction. J Oper Res Soc China. 2020;8(2):311–40.
31. Du Q, et al. Evaluation of functional magnetic resonance imaging under artificial intelligence algorithm on plan-do-check-action home nursing for patients with diabetic nephropathy. Contrast Media Mol Imaging. 2022;2022(1):9882532.
32. Menzies SW, et al. Comparison of humans versus mobile phone-powered artificial intelligence for the diagnosis and management of pigmented skin cancer in secondary care: a multicentre, prospective, diagnostic, clinical trial. Lancet Digit Health. 2023;5(10):e679–91.
33. Lipkin I, et al. Coronary CTA with AI-QCT interpretation: comparison with myocardial perfusion imaging for detection of obstructive stenosis using invasive angiography as reference standard. Am J Roentgenol. 2022;219(3):407–19.
34. Backhaus SJ, et al. Artificial intelligence fully automated myocardial strain quantification for risk stratification following acute myocardial infarction. Sci Rep. 2022;12(1):12220.
35. Sun L, et al. Exploration of the influence of early rehabilitation training on circulating endothelial progenitor cell mobilization in patients with acute ischemic stroke and its related mechanism under a lightweight artificial intelligence algorithm. Eur Rev Med Pharmacol Sci. 2023;27(12)
36. Yin H-I, et al. Combined diagnosis of multiparametric MRI-based deep learning models facilitates differentiating triple-negative breast cancer from fibroadenoma magnetic resonance BI-RADS 4 lesions. J Cancer Res Clin Oncol. 2023;149(6):2575–84.
37. Reza M, et al. Automated bone scan index as an imaging biomarker to predict overall survival in the Zometa European study/SPCG11. Eur Urol Oncol. 2021;4(1):49–55.
38. Tomaszewski MR, et al. AI-radiomics can improve inclusion criteria and clinical trial performance. Tomography. 2022;8(1):341–55.
39. Riedl S, et al. The effect of pegcetacoplan treatment on photoreceptor maintenance in geographic atrophy monitored by artificial intelligence–based OCT analysis. Ophthalmol Retina. 2022;6(11):1009–18.
40. Meng M, et al. Differentiation of breast lesions on dynamic contrast-enhanced magnetic resonance imaging (DCE-MRI) using deep transfer learning based on DenseNet201. Medicine. 2022;101(45):e31214.
41. Yang X, et al. An artificial intelligence system for distinguishing between gastrointestinal stromal tumors and leiomyomas using endoscopic ultrasonography. Endoscopy. 2022;54(03):251–61.
42. Kundisch A, et al. Deep learning algorithm in detecting intracranial hemorrhages on emergency computed tomographies. PLoS One. 2021;16(11):e0260560.
43. Esteva A, et al. A guide to deep learning in healthcare. Nat Med. 2019;25(1):24–9.
44. Nia N, Kaplanoglu E, Nasab A. Evaluation of artificial intelligence techniques in disease diagnosis and prediction. Discov Artif Intell. 2023;3:5.
45. Kumar Y, et al. Artificial intelligence in disease diagnosis: a systematic literature review, synthesizing framework and future research agenda. J Ambient Intell Humaniz Comput. 2023;14(7):8459–86.
46. Hosny A, et al. Artificial intelligence in radiology. Nat Rev Cancer. 2018;18(8):500–10.
47. Küstner T, et al. Deep-learning based super-resolution for 3D isotropic coronary MR angiography in less than a minute. Magn Reson Med. 2021;86(5):2837–52.
48. Fuin N, et al. A multi-scale variational neural network for accelerating motion-compensated whole-heart 3D coronary MR angiography. Magn Reson Imaging. 2020;70:155–67.

49. Steeden JA, et al. Rapid whole-heart CMR with single volume super-resolution. J Cardiovasc Magn Reson. 2020;22(1):56.
50. Dawes TJ, et al. Machine learning of three-dimensional right ventricular motion enables outcome prediction in pulmonary hypertension: a cardiac MR imaging study. Radiology. 2017;283(2):381–90.
51. Samad MD, et al. Predicting deterioration of ventricular function in patients with repaired tetralogy of Fallot using machine learning. Eur Heart J Cardiovasc Imaging. 2018;19(7):730–8.
52. Yang G, Yu S, Dong H, Slabaugh G, Dragotti PL, Ye X, et al. DAGAN: deep de-aliasing generative adversarial networks for fast compressed sensing MRI reconstruction. IEEE Trans Med Imaging. 2018;37(6):1310–21.
53. Bernard O, Lalande A, Zotti C, Cervenansky F, Yang X, Heng PA, et al. Deep learning techniques for automatic MRI cardiac multi-structures segmentation and diagnosis: is the problem solved? IEEE Trans Med Imaging. 2018;37(11):2514–25.
54. Khened M, Kollerathu VA, Krishnamurthi G. Fully convolutional multi-scale residual DenseNets for cardiac segmentation and automated cardiac diagnosis using ensemble of classifiers. Med Image Anal. 2019;51:21–45.
55. Tat E, Bhatt DL, Rabbat MG. Addressing bias: artificial intelligence in cardiovascular medicine. Lancet Digit Health. 2020;2(12):e635–6.
56. Herzog B, et al. Cardiovascular magnetic resonance pocket guide. Eur Soc Cardiol. 2017;
57. Schulz-Menger J, Bluemke DA, Bremerich J, Flamm SD, Fogel MA, Friedrich MG, et al. Standardized image interpretation and post-processing in cardiovascular magnetic resonance—2020 update: Society for Cardiovascular Magnetic Resonance (SCMR) Board of Trustees Task Force on standardized post-processing. J Cardiovasc Magn Reson. 2020;22(1):19.
58. Litjens G, et al. A survey on deep learning in medical image analysis. Med Image Anal. 2017;42:60–88.
59. Bernard O, et al. Deep learning techniques for automatic MRI cardiac multi-structures segmentation and diagnosis: is the problem solved? IEEE Trans Med Imaging. 2018;37(11):2514–25.
60. Litjens G, Kooi T, Bejnordi BE, Setio AAA, Ciompi F, Ghafoorian M, et al. A survey on deep learning in medical image analysis. Med Image Anal. 2017;42:60–88.
61. Pesapane F, Codari M, Sardanelli F. Artificial intelligence in medical imaging: threat or opportunity? Radiologists again at the forefront of innovation in medicine. Eur Radiol Exp. 2018;2(1):35.
62. Barberis A, Aerts H, Buffa FM. Robustness and reproducibility for AI learning in biomedical sciences: RENOIR. Sci Rep. 2024;14(1):1933.
63. Mooghali M, Stroud AM, Yoo DW, Barry BA, Grimshaw AA, Ross JS, et al. Trustworthy and ethical AI-enabled cardiovascular care: a rapid review. BMC Med Inform Decis Mak. 2024;24:247.
64. Marey A, Arjmand P, Sabe Alerab AD, Eslami MJ, Saad AM, Sanchez N, et al. Explainability, transparency and black box challenges of AI in radiology: impact on patient care in cardiovascular radiology. Egypt J Radiol Nucl Med. 2024;55:183.
65. Harishbhai Tilala M, et al. Ethical considerations in the use of artificial intelligence and machine learning in health care: a comprehensive review. Cureus. 2024;16(6):e62443.
66. Naik N, et al. Legal and ethical consideration in artificial intelligence in healthcare: who takes responsibility? Front Surg. 2022;9:862322.
67. Villegas-Martinez M, et al. The beating heart: artificial intelligence for cardiovascular application in the clinic. MAGMA. 2024;37(3):369–82.
68. Poon AIF, Sung JJY. Opening the black box of AI-medicine. J Gastroenterol Hepatol. 2021;36(3):581–4.
69. Yang G, Ye Q, Xia J. Unbox the black-box for the medical explainable AI via multi-modal and multi-Centre data fusion: a mini-review, two showcases and beyond. Inf Fusion. 2022;77:29–52.
70. Fotaki A, Puyol-Antón E, Chiribiri A, Botnar R, Pushparajah K, Prieto C. Artificial intelligence in cardiac MRI: is clinical adoption forthcoming? Front Cardiovasc Med. 2022;8:818765.
71. Fornell D. What is the ROI for adopting AI in cardiac imaging? Cardiovasc Bus. 2023;
72. Kramer CM, Barkhausen J, Flamm SD, Kim RJ, Nagel E. Standardized cardiovascular magnetic resonance imaging (CMR) protocols: 2020 update. J Cardiovasc Magn Reson. 2020;22(1):17.
73. Serruys PW, et al. Coronary computed tomographic angiography for complete assessment of coronary artery disease: JACC state-of-the-art review. J Am Coll Cardiol. 2021;78(7):713–36.
74. McCollough CH, Rajiah PS. Milestones in CT: past, present, and future. Radiology. 2023;309(1):e230803.
75. Jin L, et al. Qualitative and quantitative image analysis of 16 cm wide-coverage computed tomography compared to new-generation dual-source CT. 2020;28(3):527–39.
76. Abbara S, et al. SCCT guidelines for the performance and acquisition of coronary computed tomographic angiography: a report of the society of cardiovascular computed tomography guidelines committee: endorsed by the North American Society for Cardiovascular Imaging (NASCI). J Cardiovasc Comput Tomogr. 2016;10(6):435–49.
77. Pontone G, Baggiano A, Andreini D, Guaricci AI, Guglielmo M, Muscogiuri G, et al. Dynamic stress computed tomography perfusion with a whole-heart coverage scanner in addition to coronary computed tomography angiography for the detection of coronary artery disease: comparison with magnetic resonance imaging. JACC Cardiovasc Imaging. 2019;12(12):2460–71.

78. Lang RM, Badano LP, Mor-Avi V, Afilalo J, Armstrong A, Ernande L, et al. Recommendations for cardiac chamber quantification by echocardiography in adults: an update from the American Society of Echocardiography and the European Association of Cardiovascular Imaging. J Am Soc Echocardiogr. 2015;28(1):1–39.
79. Mor-Avi V, Lang RM, Badano LP, Belohlavek M, Cardim NM, Derumeaux G, et al. Current and evolving echocardiographic techniques for the quantitative evaluation of cardiac mechanics: ASE/EAE consensus statement on methodology and indications endorsed by the Japanese Society of Echocardiography. J Am Soc Echocardiogr. 2011;24(3):277–313.
80. Grant MD, et al. Transthoracic echocardiography: Beginner's guide with emphasis on blind spots as identified with CT and MRI. Radiographics. 2021;41(4):1022–42.
81. Slomka PJ, Berman DS, Germano G, Alexanderson E, Fish MB. Advances in SPECT and PET hardware. Prog Cardiovasc Dis. 2015;57(6):566–78.
82. Rischpler C, Nekolla SG, Dregely I, Schwaiger M. Hybrid PET/MR imaging of the heart: potential, initial experiences, and future prospects. J Nucl Med. 2013;54(3):402–15.
83. Gaemperli O, Kaufmann PA. PET and PET/CT in cardiovascular disease. Ann N Y Acad Sci. 2011;1228:109–36.
84. Nensa F, Kloth J, Tezgah E, Poeppel TD, Heusch P, Goebel J, et al. Feasibility of FDG PET/MRI in patients with cardiac sarcoidosis: first insights from a comparison of PET/CT and PET/MRI. J Nucl Med. 2014;55(12):1911–6.
85. Abbara S, Blanke P, Maroules CD, Cheezum MK, Choi AD, Han BK, et al. SCCT guidelines for the performance and acquisition of coronary computed tomographic angiography: a report of the Society of Cardiovascular Computed Tomography Guidelines Committee. J Cardiovasc Comput Tomogr. 2016;10(6):435–49.

AI-Driven Risk Stratification in Cardiology: Predicting Cardiovascular Outcomes, Sudden Cardiac Death, Cardiotoxicity, and Heart Failure with CMR

8

Amir Ghaffari Jolfayi, Sara Montazeri, Amirhossein Poopak, Amirali Soheili, Ayda Manzari Tavakoli, Alireza Salmanipour, Sara Adimi, and Kiara Rezaei-Kalantari

Abstract

Artificial Intelligence (AI) is transforming cardiovascular magnetic resonance (CMR) imaging, providing advanced tools for diagnosing and managing cardiovascular diseases. This chapter highlights AI's role in risk stratification and outcome prediction for conditions like sudden cardiac death (SCD), cardiotoxicity, and heart failure. AI innovations streamline CMR workflows by reducing scan times, managing artifacts, and automating segmentation to improve accuracy in analyzing myocardial tissue and scar quantification. Machine learning (ML) models enhance SCD prediction by integrating imaging data, such as fibrosis patterns from late gadolinium enhancement (LGE), with clinical metrics, offering more personalized risk assessments beyond traditional left ventricular ejection fraction (LVEF) criteria.

In oncology, AI-based CMR facilitates early cardiotoxicity detection by identifying subtle myocardial changes through T1/T2 mapping and radiomics. These tools enhance precision, allowing earlier intervention for patients undergoing chemotherapy. In heart failure, AI applications incorporate CMR data and electronic health records to predict hospitalizations and outcomes. Advanced radiomics combined with ML provides personalized risk models, identifying high-risk patients with superior accuracy compared to conventional methods.

While AI has revolutionized cardiovascular imaging, challenges persist, including the need for model validation across diverse populations and addressing ethical concerns like data privacy and algorithm transparency. Future directions emphasize integrating multimodal AI systems, including

Authors Amir Ghaffari Jolfayi and Sara Montazeri have contributed equality and shared the first co-authorship.

A. Ghaffari Jolfayi · S. Montazeri · A. Poopak
A. Soheili · A. Salmanipour
K. Rezaei-Kalantari (✉)
Cardiovascular Imaging Research Center, Rajaie Cardiovascular Institute, Tehran, Iran

A. Manzari Tavakoli
Student's Scientific Research Center, School of Medicine, Iran University of Medical Sciences, Tehran, Iran

S. Adimi
Cardio-Oncology Research Center, Rajaie Cardiovascular Institute, Tehran, Iran

A. Ghaffari Jolfayi (ed.), *Navigating Cardiology's Future*,
https://doi.org/10.1007/978-981-95-0313-1_8

genomic and clinical data, to refine personalized risk prediction and guide treatment strategies.

AI's integration into CMR significantly enhances diagnostic precision, risk stratification, and decision-making, making it a cornerstone for the future of cardiovascular care. This chapter explores its transformative potential and offers insights into addressing existing gaps, ensuring equitable and effective application in clinical practice.

Keywords

Cardiac magnetic resonance imaging · Deep learning · Machine learning · Artificial intelligence · Risk stratification · Cardiovascular outcomes · Sudden cardiac death · Cardiotoxicity · Heart failure

8.1 Advantages of Machine/Deep Learning in Image Acquisition, Segmentation, and Tissue Characterization

8.1.1 Acquisition Time

The application of AI in CMR has strongly affected the patient, technician, radiologist, and discovery fields. Expecting faster-streamlined scanning, AI can significantly reduce patients' time spent inside the scanner [1]. EasyScan, an AI-driven technology, has reduced technician involvement and shortened the examination time by 2 min with a nearly 12% higher signal-to-noise ratio [2].

8.1.2 Artifact Handling Through ECG Gated Image Acquisition

Moreover, images are typically acquired during the heart's resting phase using ECG gating to eliminate motion artifacts in CMR scans. However, manual identification of this optimal timing is time-consuming and may lead to incontinence. A novel deep learning system addresses this cardiac resting period detection by automatically detecting the ideal trigger point, resulting in more accurate scans, and 1 min faster than the technician [3]. Selection of the optimal inversion time (TI) for CMR scans, which is essential for detecting myocardial fibrosis, depends on the manual analysis of multiple images. AI-based tools such as convolutional neural networks automate TI selection using long–and short-term memory. This AI model analyzes the spatial and temporal resolution of TI and predicts the optimal value, achieving accuracy and matching the expert-determined TI [4]. Multichannel acquisition and non-Cartesian trajectories effectively accelerate CMR, enabling up to fivefold speedup in 2D and 3D imaging [5]. While traditional reconstruction methods, such as compressed sensing (CS)-based reconstruction, offer advantages, they are limited in computational efficiency and parameter tuning. The integration of AI-driven reconstruction algorithms in CMR is expected to improve.

8.1.3 Accurately Outlining the Boundaries

Analyzing CMR images faces challenges in accurately outlining the boundaries of heart chambers, the myocardium, and blood vessels, also known as segmentation. Also, manual segmentation methods by clinicians are required in complex regions such as the heart's trabeculae, outflow tract, apical slices, and the right ventricle, which is time-consuming and prone to errors due to variations between clinicians [6, 7]. Deep learning algorithms for automated segmentation have shown accurate results, achieving high Dice similarity coefficients [8]. For instance, Circle CVI42® (Calgary, Canada) measures cardiac function and blood flow and identifies tissue abnormalities with AI-driven contouring. CASIS (Quetigny, France) and Medviso's Segment CMR (Lund, Sweden) are mainly designed to automate quantitative and functional analyses from CMR images, leading to rapid and accurate results. Moreover, Syngo.via (Forchheim, Germany) integrates AI-driven capabilities in the automatic contouring of organs.

8.1.4 Myocardial Tissue Analysis and Scar Quantification

In an analysis of myocardial tissue, AI, particularly ML, can detect and measure the extent of myocardial scar tissue from Late Gadolinium Enhancement (LGE) CMR images [9]. Scar quantification is a valuable prognostic marker. However, LGE quantification methods lack accuracy and reproducibility, and deep learning can be integrated to address these limitations. For instance, an atlas-based approach, followed by deep neural networks, has detected fibrotic tissue in the left atrium [10]. Also, an advanced deep neural network for automatic, anatomically accurate scar segmentation from LGE images has achieved a Dice score of 0.57 compared to expert annotations. Significantly, the convolutional neural network-based approach for scar segmentation from 3D LGE-MR images has reported an average Dice score of 0.94 [11]. While these improvements demonstrate the potential of deep learning for scar segmentation, the accuracy for scar segmentation is relatively low when a U-Net-based network simultaneously segments both the myocardium and scars in hypertrophic cardiomyopathy patients [12]. Fully automated scar segmentation remains challenging due to the variability in heart motion and the unique characteristics of contrast-enhanced images in infarcted regions. Novel approaches have been explored to overcome these challenges. Non-contrast cine-CMR images instead of LGE-CMR images have been applied to assess myocardial infarction dimensions without gadolinium injection [13, 14]. For instance, a recurrent neural network from cine MR image sequences showed a high Dice score of 0.90 compared to manual annotations on LGE MR images [15].

8.1.5 Radiomics Study

Machine learning techniques proceed with high-dimensional data, contributing to the growth of radiomics, which extracts numerous quantitative features such as morphological, intensity-based, fractal-based, and texture features from images, turning them into data sets that can be analyzed with AI-based tools [16]. Texture analysis with machine learning algorithms can evaluate spatial variations and relationships between adjacent pixels, improving imaging metrics [17]. Initial applications of radiomics and tissue analysis in CMR imaging focused on the segmentation of scar tissue in myocardial infarction, improving visualization and information extraction [18]. Tissue analysis in combination with non-contrast cine and LGE imaging [19] or cine imaging alone [20] can also detect both acute and chronic infarctions and provide tissue heterogeneity data [21]. Tissue analysis can also differentiate causes of myocardial hypertrophy, such as hypertrophic cardiomyopathy, amyloidosis, and aortic stenosis [22]. Radiomics can also identify high-risk patients for fibrosis based on cine imaging [23] and provide an accurate diagnosis for myocarditis based on T1 and T2 mapping [24].

8.2 Sudden Cardiac Death (SCD) and Attributed Lethal Arrhythmias Prediction

Sudden Cardiac Death (SCD) is a global health issue, accounting for nearly six million deaths annually, with estimates suggesting that SCD comprises a notable portion of the total mortality rate in developed nations [25–27]. Lethal ventricular arrhythmias, such as ventricular tachycardia (VT) and ventricular fibrillation (VF), are the most common immediate causes of SCD, particularly in individuals with underlying ischemic heart disease and various cardiomyopathies [26–28]. Despite advancements in cardiovascular care, predicting which individuals are at risk for SCD remains a challenge.

In the United States alone, SCD claims over 300,000 lives each year, with ischemic cardiomyopathy (ICM) contributing significantly to these statistics [28–30]. Other high-risk groups include patients with hypertrophic cardiomyopathy (HCM), dilated cardiomyopathy (DCM), and arrhythmogenic cardiomyopathy (ACM), all of which carry varying degrees of arrhythmic risk [31–34].

The cornerstone of SCD prevention has traditionally been the use of implantable cardioverter-defibrillators (ICDs). However, ICDs are typically recommended based on left ventricular ejection fraction (LVEF), which, while an important predictor, does not capture the full spectrum of arrhythmic risk. Studies have shown that up to 70% of SCD cases occur in individuals with LVEF >35%, highlighting the need for more accurate risk stratification [28, 35].

8.2.1 Risk Assessment and ICD Implementation

The decision to implant an ICD for primary prevention of SCD in patients with ischemic and non-ischemic cardiomyopathy has traditionally relied on LVEF ≤35%, based on studies like MADIT II and SCD-HeFT [26, 28, 36, 37]. However, the reliance on LVEF alone is increasingly recognized as inadequate for risk prediction, as many SCD events occur in patients with preserved LVEF [28]. AI-driven models have begun to refine this process, providing more individualized risk assessments based on imaging data and clinical parameters [38]. AI models have demonstrated the ability to improve ICD decision-making by integrating complex data, including fibrosis patterns from cardiac magnetic resonance (CMR) and late gadolinium enhancement (LGE), ECG parameters, and clinical histories [26]. These models can potentially identify high-risk patients who do not meet traditional LVEF criteria for ICD implantation [35].

8.2.2 Modalities Used in SCD Risk Stratification

Electrocardiography (ECG) ECG remains a widely used tool for identifying electrical disturbances associated with increased risk of arrhythmic events. Markers such as T-wave alternans, QRS fragmentation, and heart rate variability have been studied extensively. However, their predictive power is limited when used in isolation [28].

Echocardiography Although echocardiography is essential for evaluating left ventricular function, it lacks the sensitivity to identify fibrosis and other arrhythmogenic substrates that increase SCD risk [28].

Cardiac Magnetic Resonance (CMR) CMR has emerged as a superior modality for SCD risk stratification due to its ability to identify myocardial scarring and fibrosis using LGE [39]. Fibrosis, particularly in non-ischemic cardiomyopathy, has been shown to be a powerful predictor of ventricular arrhythmias, even in patients with preserved LVEF [25, 26].

8.2.3 Use of CMR and LGE in Risk Assessment for SCD

Late gadolinium enhancement (LGE) has revolutionized the field of SCD risk prediction. LGE-CMR detects myocardial fibrosis, which acts as an arrhythmogenic focus by promoting re-entrant arrhythmias such as VT [35]. In ischemic cardiomyopathy (ICM), the peri-infarct "gray zone" identified on LGE-CMR is a significant predictor of both arrhythmias and mortality [28, 40]. In non-ischemic cardiomyopathy (NICM), the presence of mid-wall fibrosis detectable by LGE-CMR is a crucial predictor of SCD. Studies have shown that patients with even mild or moderate left ventricular dysfunction (LVEF >35%) but significant mid-wall fibrosis are at increased risk for ventricular arrhythmias [28, 35, 39]. LGE-CMR in NICM has proven more accurate than echocardiography in predicting arrhythmogenic risk, underscoring its value in risk stratification [28, 40].

8.2.4 AI-Powered CMR for Risk Assessment of SCD and Arrhythmias

The use of AI to interpret CMR data has significantly improved the accuracy of SCD risk prediction. AI algorithms can detect complex patterns in myocardial fibrosis and scar heterogeneity that may be missed by traditional analysis [26, 38, 41, 42]. In particular, machine learning models have been applied to automate the quantification of fibrosis and scar tissue, improving both sensitivity and specificity in predicting arrhythmic events [35, 41]. AI-based analysis of LGE patterns offers superior risk stratification by identifying high-risk patients based on the spatial complexity and extent of myocardial fibrosis. These models, such as those used in the DEEP RISK study, outperform conventional methods by integrating clinical data with imaging findings to offer personalized risk assessments [38]. Such AI models are particularly valuable in identifying patients who might benefit from ICD implantation, even when their LVEF is preserved [26, 35].

Radiomics and Predictive Algorithms Radiomic analysis, a technique in which advanced computational algorithms extract quantitative features from CMR images, has been utilized to assess myocardial scar heterogeneity. AI-driven radionics, particularly in patients with HCM, has proven to significantly enhance the prediction of SCD risk compared to traditional visual assessment [31, 40].

8.2.5 High-Risk Groups: ICM, DCM, HCM, ACM, and Other Cardiomyopathies

Ischemic Cardiomyopathy (ICM) In ICM patients, AI-powered CMR tools can quantify both infarct size and peri-infarct zone, which are crucial predictors of arrhythmia [28, 43]. AI-driven models that assess scar heterogeneity and quantify the degree of fibrosis have shown great promise in identifying patients at the highest risk for SCD [26, 43]. Such models provide more accurate stratification than traditional LVEF-based approaches, particularly in identifying patients who might benefit from ICDs [28, 44].

Dilated Cardiomyopathy (DCM) AI tools applied to CMR in patients with DCM allow for detailed analysis of mid-wall fibrosis. Even patients with mildly reduced LVEF but extensive mid-wall fibrosis are at significant risk for SCD, and AI can help clinicians identify these individuals with high precision [28, 35, 44].

Hypertrophic Cardiomyopathy (HCM) In HCM, fibrosis plays a key role in SCD risk. AI-based CMR analysis in HCM patients focuses on the extent and pattern of LGE, helping to refine risk stratification in this group. AI models that incorporate both fibrosis and clinical variables have proven particularly effective in predicting arrhythmic events [31, 35, 40, 44].

Arrhythmogenic Cardiomyopathy (ACM) ACM is characterized by fibrofatty replacement of the ventricular myocardium, and AI models have shown promise in stratifying risk by analyzing these abnormalities on CMR [28, 34, 45, 46]. AI tools may detect subtle patterns of ventricular changes and enhance the accuracy of SCD risk predictions in the future [26, 45, 46].

Sarcoidosis and Amyloidosis Cardiac sarcoidosis is a condition that significantly increases the risk of sudden cardiac death (SCD), primarily due to the presence of ventricular arrhythmias arising from granulomatous inflammation, myocardial fibrosis, and scarring. The heterogeneity of cardiac involvement in sarcoidosis presents challenges in predicting SCD risk, as many patients with preserved LVEF can still experience life-threatening arrhythmias [28].

Recent advances in AI and machine learning have improved the ability to predict SCD in patients with cardiac sarcoidosis by integrating multimodality imaging. A key development in this area is using a personalized two-step precision risk prediction model, which fuses CMR with positron emission tomography (PET) data. CMR with LGE is instrumental in identifying myocardial fibrosis, while PET imaging detects active inflammation [47]. In patients with cardiac sarcoidosis, fibrosis and inflammation are key predictors of SCD.

The combination of LGE-CMR findings and inflammation seen on FDG-PET has been shown to elevate the accuracy of SCD risk assessment significantly. In a recent study, AI-driven personalized heart modeling combined data from CMR and PET imaging to create a more comprehensive picture of arrhythmogenic risk. The model simulates the interaction between fibrosis and inflammation, identifying regions where these abnormalities overlap and are more likely to sustain re-entrant circuits leading to ventricular tachycardia [47]. This information, along with other clinical biomarkers, feeds into a supervised machine learning classifier, which generates a personalized risk score for each patient. This allows clinicians to predict the risk of SCD more accurately [47]. AI models such as the CHAI (Computational Heart and Artificial Intelligence) Risk Predictor help identify these high-risk areas by simulating the arrhythmic potential of the affected tissue [47].

Amyloidosis Diffuse myocardial infiltration can increase the risk of arrhythmias in amyloidosis. AI-driven imaging techniques, particularly those focusing on native T1 mapping and extracellular volume (ECV) fraction [48], offer enhanced risk prediction by identifying patients with extensive cardiac involvement [28, 49].

Improved ICD Decision-Making AI-based approaches to risk stratification offer significant advantages in guiding implantable cardioverter-defibrillator (ICD) decision-making. Traditionally, ICD implantation decisions have been based on LVEF thresholds, which do not fully capture the arrhythmogenic risk in patients with preserved LVEF but significant myocardial fibrosis or active inflammation. AI-powered models that integrate multimodal imaging allow for more precise ICD recommendations by identifying patients who may benefit from ICD therapy despite having preserved LVEF [28, 47].

Clinical Implications and Future Directions The integration of multimodal imaging with AI-based personalized heart modeling in cardiac sarcoidosis represents a major advancement in SCD risk prediction. This approach allows for better stratification of high-risk patients, reducing the likelihood of unnecessary ICD implantations and ensuring that those at the highest risk receive timely interventions [47]. The application of AI in this context holds promise for improving clinical outcomes and could be expanded to other high-risk cardiomyopathy populations [47, 50].

AI has revolutionized the integration of multiple data sources, including CMR, ECG, and clinical findings. Multimodal AI models offer comprehensive risk assessments by combining structural, electrical, and clinical data [35, 38, 51]. For instance, AI models that integrate CMR data with ECG findings have shown superior performance in identifying high-risk patients for SCD compared to conventional risk models [26, 38]. AI-driven ECG analysis can detect subtle abnormalities in electrical conduction that may correspond to underlying myocardial scarring or fibrosis. This integration allows for the early identification of arrhythmic risk, even in patients without apparent structural heart disease on imaging [26, 46].

8.3 Machine Learning and Deep Learning Applications in CMR for the Diagnosis of Cardiotoxicity

Introduction to Cardiotoxicity Cardiotoxicity broadly refers to damage to the heart muscle and its function by various chemical agents or medical treatments, mostly chemotherapeutic drugs. With the emerging rise in cancer survivorship, recognition of long-term cardiovascular complications, including chemotherapy-induced cardiotoxicity, has become a critical public health issue [52]. Epidemiologically, some reports suggest that anthracyclines (e.g., doxorubicin) can induce cardiotoxicity in up to 9–26% of treated patients, depending on dosage and patient-specific risk factors [53]. Other agents, such as trastuzumab and targeted therapies, can also lead to significant cardiac dysfunction [54]. Cardiotoxicity arises through multiple pathways, including generating free radicals, disrupting mitochondrial function, and interfering with cardiomyocyte repair processes, ultimately culminating in cellular apoptosis or necrosis [55]. From a clinical standpoint, early and accurate diagnosis of cardiotoxicity is crucial for initiating timely management [56]. Traditional diagnostic evaluations, such as echocardiography for left ventricular ejection fraction (LVEF) assessment, serum biomarkers (e.g., troponin, BNP), and electrocardiography, provide useful but sometimes limited information, especially in the subclinical stages of cardiac injury [57, 58]. Consequently, more sensitive and specific imaging modalities, such as Cardiac Magnetic Resonance (CMR), have gained traction for more refined assessments of myocardial damage [59].

The Role of CMR in Diagnosing Cardiotoxicity Cardiac Magnetic Resonance offers a comprehensive evaluation of cardiac structure and function without ionizing radiation, making it a valuable tool for repeated assessments. CMR provides highly accurate measurements of left ventricular volumes, ejection fraction, and wall thickness [60]. Beyond functional assessment, CMR-based tissue characterization techniques, such as LGE, T1 and T2 mapping, and extracellular volume (ECV) quantification, enable the identification of subtle changes in myocardial composition, such as edema, fibrosis, or infiltration [61, 62]. These parametric mapping techniques are particularly effective at detecting early myocardial injury before overt functional declines are evident on standard echocardiograms. As a result, CMR is increasingly viewed as the reference standard for diagnosing and monitoring cardiotoxicity, supporting more accurate risk stratification and decision-making regarding cardioprotective therapies [63].

Machine Learning and Deep Learning Applications in CMR for Cardiotoxicity ML encompasses algorithms that learn patterns from data to make predictions or classifications, while DL is a subset of ML that uses multi-layered neural networks capable of automatically extracting relevant features [64]. Machine learning and deep learning methods in CMR enable rapid, consistent, and reproducible analysis of imaging data for tasks like segmentation, disease classification, and outcome prediction, surpassing traditional manual or rule-based approaches in detecting and monitoring cardiotoxicity [65].

In a recent study addressing automated CMR analysis for cardiotoxicity evaluation, researchers leveraged Displacement Encoding with Stimulated Echoes (DENSE) MRI to measure LV strain, an early indicator of breast cancer chemotherapy-induced cardiac damage [66]. Their approach combined a custom DeepLabV3+ deep convolutional neural network (DCNN) with a ResNet-50 backbone to segment LV chambers in 42 breast cancer patient datasets. The segmented images were used for automated LV chamber quantification (e.g., LV end-diastolic diameter, ejection fraction) and radial strain calculations via the Radial Point Interpolation Method (RPIM). Segmentation accuracy reached 97%, with a Dice coefficient of 0.89. Cronbach's Alpha correlation (C-Alpha = 0.97) further confirmed the strong agreement between DENSE-derived and SSFP-derived ejection fractions, as well as a vendor-based method. These findings underscore the feasibility of integrating DCNN-based segmentation into DENSE CMR workflows to enhance automated strain analysis and improve early detection of cardiotoxicity in breast cancer patients.

In a recent investigation of HER2-positive breast cancer patients undergoing trastuzumab therapy, researchers evaluated subclinical cardiotoxicity by comparing CMR- and speckle tracking echocardiography (2DE-ST)-derived global longitudinal and radial strains (GLS/GRS) [67]. Although CMR is considered the gold standard for cardiac function assessment, it remains underutilized for routine monitoring. Instead, the authors demonstrated that 2DE-ST could serve as a feasible alternative for early detection, particularly by incorporating changes in strain measurements over time. Notably, they found only weak correlations between 2DE-ST and CMR GLS/GRS; however, strain parameters measured at 3 months predicted subsequent reductions in CMR-derived LVEF and were strongly linked to later cardiotoxicity. While this study did not incorporate an ML or DL framework, it highlights how quantitative strain parameters—whether measured via CMR or echocardiography—could be integrated into ML/DL pipelines in future research to enhance early cardiotoxicity prediction, optimize patient monitoring, and improve clinical decision-making.

A recent study of 48 oncology patients assessed the precision of fully automated AI-based analysis versus expert human readers in evaluating LVEF and global longitudinal strain (GLS) using both echocardiography (TTE) and CMR [68]. While TTE-based AI performed comparably to human analysis for LVEF, human measurements remained superior for GLS. Notably, for CMR images, where no analysis failures occurred, AI-based methods outperformed expert readers in LVEF measurement precision, underscoring the modality's robust image quality and the emerging advantages of AI in this setting. These findings reinforce that continued development of fully automated algorithms can enhance monitoring for chemotherapy-related cardiac dysfunction (CTRCD), ultimately offering improved accuracy, reproducibility, and confidence in cardiotoxicity surveillance protocols for cancer patients.

A recent prospective study by Talebi et al. investigated an ML-based radiomics approach to predict treatment-induced cardiotoxicity in left-sided breast cancer patients [69]. Although the researchers employed echocardiography as their primary imaging modality, their workflow and findings are highly relevant to the broader use of CMR in cardiotoxicity assessment. First, they extracted a comprehensive set of dosimetric, demographic, clinical, and imaging (radiomics) features from ultrasound data and combined these variables in ML models to classify patients at high risk for cardiotoxicity. Their key innovation lay in using radionics-derived textural features—typically too subtle for conventional image interpretation—to enhance predictive accuracy, with the area under the ROC curve values reaching up to 97%. Translating this approach to CMR would be straightforward: CMR's superior spatial and tissue characterization capabilities would further refine the radiomics feature space, potentially boosting model performance for early detection of subclinical cardiotoxic changes. Ultimately, this work underscores how integrating ML-driven radiomics with multiparametric imaging can lead to more sensitive, personalized risk stratification for patients at risk of cardiotoxicity.

In conclusion, the integration of CMR imaging with advanced ML and DL techniques holds immense promise for improving the early detection and monitoring of cardiotoxicity in cancer patients. While conventional diagnostic tools (e.g., echocardiography, serum biomarkers) remain integral to clinical practice, CMR provides unparalleled precision in quantifying cardiac function and tissue changes—capabilities now enhanced by automated segmentation, radiomics-based texture analysis, and predictive modeling. Studies leveraging ML/DL pipelines have demonstrated superior performance in both image interpretation and risk stratification, especially when combining imaging data with clinical, demographic, and dosimetric parameters. As these algorithms mature and become more widely adopted, clinicians will be able to detect subtle myocardial injuries earlier, customize surveillance intervals, and personalize therapeutic strategies, ultimately reducing long-term cardiac complications in oncology populations.

8.4 Machine Learning and Deep Learning Applications in CMR for Diagnosis and Prognosis Stratification in Heart Failure

The lifetime risk of developing HF is estimated at 24%, meaning nearly one in four individuals will experience HF during their lifetime [70]. Globally, the proportion of patients with HF and preserved ejection fraction (HFpEF) is increasing, yet outcomes remain poor despite advancements in treatment options [71, 72].

HF is among the costliest healthcare conditions to manage in high-income countries [73]. Patients often undergo extensive diagnostic tests, invasive procedures, and therapies throughout the progression of their illness [74]. This generates vast data, typically consolidated into registries or institutional databases [75]. These datasets are valuable for assessing healthcare utilization, care quality, costs, and disease progression. However, the sheer volume, complexity, and dynamic nature of this "big data" pose significant challenges for traditional analytical methods to interpret effectively.

Several factors hinder the appropriate care of each patient in HF, including diagnostic uncertainty, variability in treatment outcomes, and safety responses due to the limited generalizability of clinical trial findings, challenges in risk stratification, and insufficient integration of data at the point of care. Machine learning (ML) offers significant potential to address these HF challenges, providing advantages surpassing traditional human-derived models [73].

Cardiovascular magnetic resonance (CMR) imaging has become a standard diagnostic and management tool for systolic heart failure [76]. Its widespread use is supported by its ability to deliver a comprehensive set of phenotypic markers [77–79]. These markers effectively differentiate between ischemic and non-ischemic causes, assess tissue injury patterns, detect valvular issues, and provide gold-standard measurements for chamber volumes, ventricular function, and mass [76, 80].

8.4.1 ML and DL in Heart Failure Outcome Prediction

Several studies have investigated the diagnosis and prognosis of heart failure through the integration of machine and deep learning in CMR imaging. Cornhill et al. [76] developed and validated an innovative risk model for predicting time to HF hospitalization on a patient-specific basis by incorporating routinely reported CMR variables, patient-reported health status, and electronic health records. The study excluded patients with conditions like cardiac amyloid, sarcoidosis, hypertrophic cardiomyopathy, or acute cardiomyopathy states to ensure a homogeneous cohort, resulting in a dataset of 1775 patients with reduced systolic function (LVEF $\leq$50%) confirmed through CMR imaging. Standardized protocols captured ventricular volumes, function, and fibrosis patterns, with quantitative analysis performed using validated software. The study developed two risk models: a machine learning (ML) model based on Random Survival Forest (RSF) and a competing risk Fine-Gray model (FGM). The ML model used 15 variables, including CMR metrics (e.g., LVESVi, RVEDVi, LVEF) and late gadolinium enhancement (LGE) patterns, while the FGM model was optimized through univariable analysis and backward variable selection. ML-based RSF model achieved a C-index of 0.77 and AUC values of 0.87, 0.83, and 0.80 for 90-day, 1-year, and 2-year predictions, identifying high-risk patients with significantly increased HF hospitalization rates. The FGM model demonstrated similar performance with a C-index of 0.77 and comparable AUC values.

More recently, Pujadas et al. [81] aimed to evaluate the feasibility of using CMR radionics combined with machine learning techniques to predict incident atrial fibrillation (AF), HF, myocardial infarction (MI), and stroke. Participants with incident AF, HF, MI, or stroke during longitudinal follow-up were included in the study. Data collected for each participant comprised vascular risk factors (VRFs), CMR indices, and CMR images. Three regions of interest were segmented: the right ventricle cavity, left ventricle cavity, and LV myocardium, assessed during both end-systole and end-diastole phases. Radiomics features were extracted from the 3D volumes of these regions. Seven machine learning models were developed for each cardiovascular disease (CVD), incorporating VRFs, CMR indices, and radiomics features individually and in combination. A support vector machine classifier was used, and performance metrics such as accuracy, sensitivity, specificity, and area under the curve (AUC) were reported.

In this study, HF prediction showed the most significant improvement when CMR indices were included (VRF + CMR + Rad: accuracy

0.79, AUC 0.84). Notably, combining only VRFs and radiomics (VRF + Rad) yielded nearly equivalent results (accuracy 0.77, AUC 0.83), underscoring the potential of integrating radiomics features with VRFs and CMR indices for enhanced predictive modeling of cardiovascular diseases.

Ambale-Venkatesh et al. [82] evaluated the effectiveness of Random Survival Forests (RSF), a machine learning method, in predicting six cardiovascular outcomes compared to traditional risk scores, using data from 6814 participants in the Multi-Ethnic Study of Atherosclerosis (MESA). They tested nine predictive models, leveraging RSF for variable selection based on mean minimal depth and comparing them with Cox regression-based methods, such as LASSO-Cox and AIC-Cox. RSF demonstrated strong performance in prediction and variable selection, outperforming traditional methods in many cases. Using RSF to identify the top 20 predictors (RSF-20) enhanced the efficiency of refined Cox regression models, which achieved high C-indices and low Brier Scores, comparable to RSF-20. Notably, RSF-20 outperformed the MESA HF15 risk score in predicting heart failure (C-index: 0.80, BS: 0.038). Key predictors included elevated NT-proBNP, increased LV volume, and reduced LV function via MRI, highlighting RSF's potential in improving cardiovascular risk prediction.

8.5 Future Directions and Knowledge Gaps

The future of AI in SCD risk assessment lies in personalized risk models that incorporate a wide range of data points, including genomic information, biomarkers, and advanced imaging findings [26, 28, 83]. AI models can provide real-time, individualized risk predictions that evolve as new clinical data becomes available, offering a dynamic approach to patient management [26, 35, 84]. While AI models show promise, validation across diverse populations and clinical settings is critical. Current AI models must be tested in larger, multi-center trials to ensure their generalizability and to address concerns regarding potential biases in algorithmic decision-making [28, 85].

As AI becomes more integrated into clinical workflows, ethical concerns such as data privacy, algorithm transparency, and the role of AI in clinical decision-making must be addressed. The need for clear regulatory frameworks and clinician oversight remains paramount as AI-driven tools gain more widespread adoption [28, 35, 86].

AI is transforming risk stratification by enhancing the predictive power of cardiac imaging, particularly by using CMR and LGE. By detecting arrhythmic substrates such as myocardial fibrosis with greater accuracy, AI-powered models offer a personalized approach to identifying high-risk patients. These advancements significantly impact ICD decision-making, allowing clinicians to move beyond traditional LVEF-based risk models. While the future of AI in this field is promising, further research is needed to validate these models and integrate them into routine clinical practice [26, 28, 35, 84].

References

1. Villegas-Martinez M, de Villedon de Naide V, Muthurangu V, Bustin A. The beating heart: artificial intelligence for cardiovascular application in the clinic. MAGMA. 2024;37(3):369–82.
2. Edalati M, Zheng Y, Watkins MP, Chen J, Liu L, Zhang S, et al. Implementation and prospective clinical validation of AI-based planning and shimming techniques in cardiac MRI. Med Phys. 2022;49(1):129–43.
3. Wood G, Pedersen AU, Kunze KP, Neji R, Hajhosseiny R, Wetzl J, et al. Automated detection of cardiac rest period for trigger delay calculation for image-based navigator coronary magnetic resonance angiography. J Cardiovasc Magn Reson. 2023;25(1):52.
4. Bahrami N, Retson T, Blansit K, Wang K, Hsiao A. Automated selection of myocardial inversion time with a convolutional neural network: spatial temporal ensemble myocardium inversion network (STEMI-NET). Magn Reson Med. 2019;81(5):3283–91.
5. Bustin A, Fuin N, Botnar RM, Prieto C. From compressed-sensing to artificial intelligence-based

cardiac MRI reconstruction. Front Cardiovasc Med. 2020;7:501814.
6. Suinesiaputra A, Bluemke DA, Cowan BR, Friedrich MG, Kramer CM, Kwong R, et al. Quantification of LV function and mass by cardiovascular magnetic resonance: multi-center variability and consensus contours. J Cardiovasc Magn Reson. 2015;17:1–8.
7. Lundervold AS, Lundervold A. An overview of deep learning in medical imaging focusing on MRI. Z Med Phys. 2019;29(2):102–27.
8. Bernard O, Lalande A, Zotti C, Cervenansky F, Yang X, Heng P-A, et al. Deep learning techniques for automatic MRI cardiac multi-structures segmentation and diagnosis: is the problem solved? IEEE Trans Med Imaging. 2018;37(11):2514–25.
9. Kim RJ, Fieno DS, Parrish TB, Harris K, Chen E-L, Simonetti O, et al. Relationship of MRI delayed contrast enhancement to irreversible injury, infarct age, and contractile function. Circulation. 1999;100(19):1992–2002.
10. Yang G, Zhuang X, Khan H, Haldar S, Nyktari E, Li L, et al. Fully automatic segmentation and objective assessment of atrial scars for long-standing persistent atrial fibrillation patients using late gadolinium-enhanced MRI. Med Phys. 2018;45(4):1562–76.
11. Zabihollahy F, White JA, Ukwatta E. Convolutional neural network-based approach for segmentation of left ventricle myocardial scar from 3D late gadolinium enhancement MR images. Med Phys. 2019;46(4):1740–51.
12. Fahmy AS, Rausch J, Neisius U, Chan RH, Maron MS, Appelbaum E, et al. Automated cardiac MR scar quantification in hypertrophic cardiomyopathy using deep convolutional neural networks. JACC Cardiovasc Imaging. 2018;11(12):1917–8.
13. Zhang Q, Burrage MK, Shanmuganathan M, Gonzales RA, Lukaschuk E, Thomas KE, et al. Artificial intelligence for contrast-free MRI: scar assessment in myocardial infarction using deep learning–based virtual native enhancement. Circulation. 2022;146(20):1492–503.
14. Avard E, Shiri I, Hajianfar G, Abdollahi H, Kalantari KR, Houshmand G, et al. Non-contrast cine cardiac magnetic resonance image radiomics features and machine learning algorithms for myocardial infarction detection. Comput Biol Med. 2022;141:105145.
15. Xu C, Xu L, Gao Z, Zhao S, Zhang H, Zhang Y, et al. Direct delineation of myocardial infarction without contrast agents using a joint motion feature learning architecture. Med Image Anal. 2018;50:82–94.
16. Gillies RJ, Kinahan PE, Hricak H. Radiomics: images are more than pictures, they are data. Radiology. 2016;278(2):563–77.
17. Baessler B, Mannil M, Oebel S, Maintz D, Alkadhi H, Manka R. Subacute and chronic left ventricular myocardial scar: accuracy of texture analysis on nonenhanced cine MR images. Radiology. 2018;286(1):103–12.
18. Kotu LP, Engan K, Skretting K, Måløy F, Ørn S, Woie L, et al. Probability mapping of scarred myocardium using texture and intensity features in CMR images. Biomed Eng Online. 2013;12:1–19.
19. Larroza A, Materka A, López-Lereu MP, Monmeneu JV, Bodí V, Moratal D. Differentiation between acute and chronic myocardial infarction by means of texture analysis of late gadolinium enhancement and cine cardiac magnetic resonance imaging. Eur J Radiol. 2017;92:78–83.
20. Zhang N, Yang G, Gao Z, Xu C, Zhang Y, Shi R, et al. Deep learning for diagnosis of chronic myocardial infarction on nonenhanced cardiac cine MRI. Radiology. 2019;291(3):606–17.
21. Beliveau P, Cheriet F, Anderson SA, Taylor JL, Arai AE, Hsu L-Y. Quantitative assessment of myocardial fibrosis in an age-related rat model by ex vivo late gadolinium enhancement magnetic resonance imaging with histopathological correlation. Comput Biol Med. 2015;65:103–13.
22. Thornhill RE, Cocker M, Dwivedi G, Dennie C, Fuller L, Dick A, et al. Quantitative texture features as objective metrics of enhancement heterogeneity in hypertrophic cardiomyopathy. J Cardiovasc Magn Reson. 2014;16:1–2.
23. Pu C, Hu X, Lv S, Wu Y, Yu F, Zhu W, et al. Identification of fibrosis in hypertrophic cardiomyopathy: a radiomic study on cardiac magnetic resonance cine imaging. Eur Radiol. 2023;33(4):2301–11.
24. Baessler B, Luecke C, Lurz J, Klingel K, Von Roeder M, De Waha S, et al. Cardiac MRI texture analysis of T1 and T2 maps in patients with infarctlike acute myocarditis. Radiology. 2018;289(2):357–65.
25. Holmstrom L, Chugh H, Nakamura K, Bhanji Z, Seifer M, Uy-Evanado A, et al. An ECG-based artificial intelligence model for assessment of sudden cardiac death risk. Commun Med. 2024;4(1):17.
26. Stephens K. Machine learning predicts risk of death in patients with suspected or known heart disease. AXIS Imaging News. 2021;
27. Mehra R. Global public health problem of sudden cardiac death. J Electrocardiol. 2007;40(6, Supplement 1):S118-S22
28. Zaman S, Goldberger JJ, Kovoor P. Sudden death risk-stratification in 2018–2019: the old and the new. Heart Lung Circ. 2019;28(1):57–64.
29. Kuriachan VP, Sumner GL, Mitchell LB. Sudden cardiac death. Curr Probl Cardiol. 2015;40(4):133–200.
30. Al-Zaiti SS, Fallavollita JA, Canty JM Jr, Carey MG. Electrocardiographic predictors of sudden and non-sudden cardiac death in patients with ischemic cardiomyopathy. Heart Lung. 2014;43(6):527–33.
31. Fahmy AS, Rowin EJ, Jaafar N, Chan RH, Rodriguez J, Nakamori S, et al. Radiomics of late gadolinium enhancement reveals prognostic value of myocardial scar heterogeneity in hypertrophic cardiomyopathy. Cardiovasc Imaging. 2024;17(1):16–27.

32. O'Mahony C, Elliott P, McKenna W. Sudden cardiac death in hypertrophic cardiomyopathy. Circ Arrhythm Electrophysiol. 2013;6(2):443–51.
33. Grimm W, Maisch B. Sudden cardiac death in dilated cardiomyopathy–therapeutic options. Herz. 2002;27(8):750–9.
34. Cadrin-Tourigny J, Bosman LP, Wang W, Tadros R, Bhonsale A, Bourfiss M, et al. Sudden cardiac death prediction in arrhythmogenic right ventricular cardiomyopathy: a multinational collaboration. Circ Arrhythm Electrophysiol. 2021;14(1):e008509.
35. Holmström L, Zhang FZ, Ouyang D, Dey D, Slomka PJ, Chugh SS. Artificial intelligence in ventricular arrhythmias and sudden death. Arrhythm Electrophysiol Rev. 2023:12.
36. Adabag S, Patton KK, Buxton AE, Rector TS, Ensrud KE, Vakil K, et al. Association of implantable cardioverter defibrillators with survival in patients with and without improved ejection fraction: secondary analysis of the sudden cardiac death in heart failure trial. JAMA Cardiol. 2017;2(7):767–74.
37. Gula LJ, Klein GJ, Hellkamp AS, Massel D, Krahn AD, Skanes AC, et al. Ejection fraction assessment and survival: an analysis of the sudden cardiac death in heart failure trial (SCD-HeFT). Am Heart J. 2008;156(6):1196–200.
38. Kolk MZ, Ruipérez-Campillo S, Allaart CP, Wilde AA, Knops RE, Narayan SM, et al. Multimodal explainable artificial intelligence identifies patients with non-ischaemic cardiomyopathy at risk of lethal ventricular arrhythmias. Sci Rep. 2024;14(1):14889.
39. Li Y, Xu Y, Li W, Guo J, Wan K, Wang J, et al. Cardiac MRI to predict sudden cardiac death risk in dilated cardiomyopathy. Radiology. 2023;307(3):e222552.
40. Wang J, Yang S, Ma X, Zhao K, Yang K, Yu S, et al. Assessment of late gadolinium enhancement in hypertrophic cardiomyopathy improves risk stratification based on current guidelines. Eur Heart J. 2023;44(45):4781–92.
41. Xie E, Sung E, Saad E, Trayanova N, Wu KC, Chrispin J. Advanced imaging for risk stratification for ventricular arrhythmias and sudden cardiac death. Front Cardiovasc Med. 2022;9:884767.
42. GhaffariJolfayi A, Salmanipour A, Heshmat-Ghahdarijani K, MozafaryBazargany M, Azimi A, Pirouzi P, et al. Machine learning-based interpretation of non-contrast feature tracking strain analysis and T1/T2 mapping for assessing myocardial viability. Sci Rep. 2025;15(1):753.
43. Popescu DM, Shade JK, Lai C, Aronis KN, Ouyang D, Moorthy MV, et al. Arrhythmic sudden death survival prediction using deep learning analysis of scarring in the heart. Nat Cardiovasc Res. 2022;1(4):334–43.
44. Guo J, Lu H, Chen Y, Zeng M, Jin H. Artificial intelligence study on left ventricular function among normal individuals, hypertrophic cardiomyopathy and dilated cardiomyopathy patients using 1.5 T cardiac cine MR images obtained by SSFP sequence. Br J Radiol. 2022;95(1133):20201060
45. Villuendas R, Kadish AH. Cardiac magnetic resonance for risk stratification: the sudden death risk portrayed. Prog Cardiovasc Dis. 2008;51(2):128–34.
46. Haq IU, Liu K, Giudicessi JR, Siontis KC, Asirvatham SJ, Attia ZI, et al. Artificial intelligence-enhanced electrocardiogram for arrhythmogenic right ventricular cardiomyopathy detection. Eur Heart J Digit Health. 2024;5(2):192–4.
47. Shade JK, Prakosa A, Popescu DM, Yu R, Okada DR, Chrispin J, et al. Predicting risk of sudden cardiac death in patients with cardiac sarcoidosis using multimodality imaging and personalized heart modeling in a multivariable classifier. Science. Advances. 2021;7(31):eabi8020
48. Oikonomou EK, Sangha V, Vasisht Shankar S, Coppi A, Krumholz H, Nasir K, et al. Tracking the preclinical progression of transthyretin amyloid cardiomyopathy using artificial intelligence-enabled electrocardiography and echocardiography. medRxiv. 2024;2024.08. 25.24312556
49. Ahmadi-Hadad A, De Rosa E, Di Serafino L, Esposito G. Artificial intelligence as a tool for diagnosis of cardiac amyloidosis: a systematic review. J Med Biol Eng. 2024:1–15.
50. Franke KB, Marshall H, Kennewell P, Pham H-D, Tully PJ, Rattanakosit T, et al. Risk and predictors of sudden death in cardiac sarcoidosis: a systematic review and meta-analysis. Int J Cardiol. 2021;328:130–40.
51. Jaltotage B, Lu J, Dwivedi G. Use of artificial intelligence including multimodal systems to improve the management of cardiovascular disease. Can J Cardiol. 2024;
52. Ewer MS, Ewer SM. Cardiotoxicity of anticancer treatments. Nat Rev Cardiol. 2015;12(9):547–58.
53. Lotrionte M, Biondi-Zoccai G, Abbate A, Lanzetta G, D'Ascenzo F, Malavasi V, et al. Review and meta-analysis of incidence and clinical predictors of anthracycline cardiotoxicity. Am J Cardiol. 2013;112(12):1980–4.
54. Keefe DL. Trastuzumab-associated cardiotoxicity. Cancer. 2002;95(7):1592–600.
55. Rawat PS, Jaiswal A, Khurana A, Bhatti JS, Navik U. Doxorubicin-induced cardiotoxicity: an update on the molecular mechanism and novel therapeutic strategies for effective management. Biomed Pharmacother. 2021;139:111708.
56. Kubota S, Hara H, Hiroi Y. Current status and future perspectives of onco-cardiology: importance of early detection and intervention for cardiotoxicity, and cardiovascular complication of novel cancer treatment. Global Health Med. 2021;3(4):214–25.
57. Cocco L, Chiaparini A, Saffi M, Leiria T. Global longitudinal strain for the early detection of chemotherapy-induced cardiotoxicity: a systematic review and meta-analysis. Clin Oncol. 2022;34(8):514–25.

58. Díaz-Antón B, Madurga R, Zorita B, Wasniewski S, Moreno-Arciniegas A, López-Melgar B, et al. Early detection of anthracycline-and trastuzumab-induced cardiotoxicity: value and optimal timing of serum biomarkers and echocardiographic parameters. ESC Heart Failure. 2022;9(2):1127–37.
59. Giusca S, Korosoglou G, Montenbruck M, Geršak B, Schwarz AK, Esch S, et al. Multiparametric early detection and prediction of cardiotoxicity using myocardial strain, T1 and T2 mapping, and biochemical markers: a longitudinal cardiac resonance imaging study during 2 years of follow-up. Circulation. Cardiovasc Imaging. 2021;14(6):e012459.
60. Xu J, Yang W, Zhao S, Lu M. State-of-the-art myocardial strain by CMR feature tracking: clinical applications and future perspectives. Eur Radiol. 2022;32(8):5424–35.
61. Meier C, Eisenblätter M, Gielen S. Myocardial late gadolinium enhancement (LGE) in cardiac magnetic resonance imaging (CMR)—an important risk marker for cardiac disease. J Cardiovasc Dev Dis. 2024;11(2):40.
62. Thongsongsang R, Songsangjinda T, Tanapibunpon P, Krittayaphong R. Native T1 mapping and extracellular volume fraction for differentiation of myocardial diseases from normal CMR controls in routine clinical practice. BMC Cardiovasc Disord. 2021;21(1):270.
63. Houbois CP, Nolan M, Somerset E, Shalmon T, Esmaeilzadeh M, Lamacie MM, et al. Serial cardiovascular magnetic resonance strain measurements to identify cardiotoxicity in breast cancer: comparison with echocardiography. Cardiovasc Imaging. 2021;14(5):962.
64. Janiesch C, Zschech P, Heinrich K. Machine learning and deep learning. Electron Mark. 2021;31(3):685–95.
65. Minaee S, Boykov Y, Porikli F, Plaza A, Kehtarnavaz N, Terzopoulos D. Image segmentation using deep learning: A survey. IEEE Trans Pattern Anal Mach Intell. 2021;44(7):3523–42.
66. Kar J, Cohen MV, McQuiston SP, Malozzi CM. A deep-learning semantic segmentation approach to fully automated MRI-based left-ventricular deformation analysis in cardiotoxicity. Magn Reson Imaging. 2021;78:127–39.
67. Bouwer N, Liesting C, Kofflard M, Brugts J, Kock M, Kitzen J, et al. 2D-echocardiography vs cardiac MRI strain using deep learning: a prospective cohort study in patients with HER2-positive breast cancer undergoing trastuzumab. Eur Heart J Cardiovasc Imaging. 2021;22(Suppl 1):jeaa356.
68. Dowsing B, Ioannou A, Menacho K, Culotta V, Bhuva A, Ferreira A, et al. Comparison of the accuracy and reproducibility of AI based echocardiography and CMR analysis for cardiac function assessment in oncology patients at risk of cardiotoxicity. Eur Heart J Cardiovasc Imaging. 2023;24(Suppl 1):jead119.
69. Talebi A, Bitarafan-Rajabi A, Alizadeh-asl A, Seilani P, Khajetash B, Hajianfar G, et al. Machine learning based radiomics model to predict radiotherapy induced cardiotoxicity in breast cancer. J Appl Clin Med Phys. 2024:e14614.
70. Bozkurt B, Ahmad T, Alexander KM, Baker WL, Bosak K, Breathett K, et al. Heart failure epidemiology and outcomes statistics: A report of the Heart Failure Society of America. J Card Fail. 2023;29(10):1412–51.
71. Tromp J, Ferreira JP, Janwanishstaporn S, Shah M, Greenberg B, Zannad F, et al. Heart failure around the world. Eur J Heart Fail. 2019;21(10):1187–96.
72. Pieske B, Tschöpe C, de Boer RA, Fraser AG, Anker SD, Donal E, et al. How to diagnose heart failure with preserved ejection fraction: the HFA-PEFF diagnostic algorithm: a consensus recommendation from the heart failure association (HFA) of the European Society of Cardiology (ESC). Eur Heart J. 2019;40(40):3297–317.
73. Averbuch T, Sullivan K, Sauer A, Mamas MA, Voors AA, Gale CP, et al. Applications of artificial intelligence and machine learning in heart failure. Eur Heart J Digit Health. 2022;3(2):311–22.
74. Cook JA, Collins GS. The rise of big clinical databases. Br J Surg. 2015;102(2):e93–e101.
75. Docherty AB, Lone NI. Exploiting big data for critical care research. Curr Opin Crit Care. 2015;21(5):467–72.
76. Cornhill AK, Dykstra S, Satriano A, Labib D, Mikami Y, Flewitt J, et al. Machine learning patient-specific prediction of heart failure hospitalization using cardiac MRI-based phenotype and electronic health information. Front Cardiovasc Med. 2022;9:890904.
77. Mordi I, Bezerra H, Carrick D, Tzemos N. The combined incremental prognostic value of LVEF, late gadolinium enhancement, and global circumferential strain assessed by CMR. JACC Cardiovasc Imaging. 2015;8(5):540–9.
78. McCrohon JA, Moon JC, Prasad SK, McKenna WJ, Lorenz CH, Coats AJ, et al. Differentiation of heart failure related to dilated cardiomyopathy and coronary artery disease using gadolinium-enhanced cardiovascular magnetic resonance. Circulation. 2003;108(1):54–9.
79. Stirrat J, White JA. The prognostic role of late gadolinium enhancement magnetic resonance imaging in patients with cardiomyopathy. Can J Cardiol. 2013;29(3):329–36.
80. Gajjar K, Kashyap K, Badlani J, Williams RB, Biederman RWW. A review of the pivotal role of cardiac MRI in mitral valve regurgitation. Echocardiography. 2021;38(1):128–41.
81. Pujadas ER, Raisi-Estabragh Z, Szabo L, McCracken C, Morcillo CI, Campello VM, et al. Prediction of incident cardiovascular events using machine learning and CMR radiomics. Eur Radiol. 2023;33(5):3488–500.

82. Ambale-Venkatesh B, Yang X, Wu CO, Liu K, Hundley WG, McClelland R, et al. Cardiovascular event prediction by machine learning. Circ Res. 2017;121(9):1092–101.
83. Haq I-U, Haq I, Xu B. Artificial intelligence in personalized cardiovascular medicine and cardiovascular imaging. Cardiovasc Diagn Ther. 2021;11(3):911.
84. Aqel S, Syaj S, Al-Bzour A, Abuzanouneh F, Al-Bzour N, Ahmad J. Artificial intelligence and machine learning applications in sudden cardiac arrest prediction and management: a comprehensive review. Curr Cardiol Rep. 2023;25(11):1391–6.
85. Mahmood U, Shukla-Dave A, Chan H-P, Drukker K, Samala RK, Chen Q, et al. Artificial intelligence in medicine: mitigating risks and maximizing benefits via quality assurance, quality control, and acceptance testing. BJR|. Artif Intell. 2024;1(1):ubae003
86. Safdar NM, Banja JD, Meltzer CC. Ethical considerations in artificial intelligence. Eur J Radiol. 2020;122:108768.

Correction to: SWOT Analysis of the Integration of MRI in Cardiology: Strengths, Weaknesses, Opportunities, and Threats

Amir Ghaffari Jolfayi, Mahshad Sarikhani,
Aryan Aarabi, Hamidreza Ghasemirad,
Zahra Dehghanian,
and Mohammadhossein Mozafarybazargany

Correction to:
Chapter 7 in: A. Ghaffari Jolfayi (ed.), *Navigating Cardiology's Future*, https://doi.org/10.1007/978-981-95-0313-1_7

This book was inadvertently published with the incorrect author name Mhashad Sarikhani and the affiliation has been updated for this chapter. The initially published version has now been corrected.

The updated version of this chapter can be found at
https://doi.org/10.1007/978-981-95-0313-1_7

A. Ghaffari Jolfayi (ed.), *Navigating Cardiology's Future*,
https://doi.org/10.1007/978-981-95-0313-1_9

MIX
Papier aus verantwortungsvollen Quellen
Paper from responsible sources
FSC® C105338

If you have any concerns about our products,
you can contact us on
ProductSafety@springernature.com

In case Publisher is established outside the EU,
the EU authorized representative is:
Springer Nature Customer Service Center GmbH
Europaplatz 3, 69115 Heidelberg, Germany

Printed by Libri Plureos GmbH
in Hamburg, Germany